Finding Kali

Also by Kali Rae Wheeler

Losing Kali
Missing Kali

Book 3 of the Finding Kali Trilogy

Finding Kali

Synchronicity in the 6 and Learning to Swim Good

Kali Rae Wheeler

ISBN: 978-1629670980
Library of Congress Control Number: 2017942559

This book is dedicated to the people struggling with either a mental disorder or a pseudo-mental disorder fueled by Big Pharma, abuse, or trauma, and to anyone who's ever been a victim of sexual assault or sexual misconduct in the workplace and to any soul who's been struck by the increase in mass shootings around the nation and our world.

We are all in this together.

Love and light to you.

XO Kali Rae

Contents

Book 3

Finding Kali

Preface

[DISCLAMER: Same Info as *Losing Kali* & *Missing Kali*]

Seven years from the time my pharmaceutical hell commenced, I found myself in a frenzied search for answers. I was past the point of realizing what had happened to me and was now out for justice. It was time to become the detective of my past and place the pieces of this catastrophic jigsaw puzzle back together. I needed to collect information outside of my experiences. I found myself reeling from the pain surfacing from all the self-excavation. I needed the inspiration to press forward; to continue past how much I wanted to pull my hair out and burn the doctor's records.

I found a few documentaries while working late night in the recording studio, which provided a spark of perseverance and the validity to continue climbing the mountain toward the summit. A clear pattern was emerging; the things that I experienced were not unique to me, they were plaguing the nation, even if it was behind closed doors. There was a real bad ass monster that I needed to slay for the rest of us. One documentary, in particular, *Boy Interrupted* (Perry 2009), clarified a critical concept and emblazoned it into my mind.

The documentary is about a teenage boy who suffered from bipolar disorder. He showed signs as early as two years old. He had dramatic mood swings where he said violent things. He would isolate himself. He would throw tantrums. All the typical mental illness checkmarks were there. He was also very well-liked and had many friends.

After weaning himself off of his prescriptions due to their adverse side effects; feeling tired, numb, headachy, etc., that he had reportedly (by parents, teachers, and friends) been doing so well on, he tragically took his own life.

What shook me to the core was what he had written on his laptop just moments before. He wrote of the universal emotions that plague the process of growing up. They were emotions that I had documented clearly, but more importantly, remembered clearly, and felt so profoundly. The catch is that I reported feeling these things more powerfully while under the influence of psychotropic drugs.

My lack of self-awareness and the inability to control impulses came out of thin air. I may have felt the same things no matter what, but when I was on the drugs, the desire to act was tangible. Many times I felt like I was being drawn to the edge of the cliff or taunted by the pill bottle to take more. I can still, to this day, remember the unmistakable surge of adrenaline that accompanied these feelings. It was animalistic: the feeling similar to sprinting the last quarter-mile of a 5k marathon using some strength and speed I never knew I had.

The impulses were often so intense that I had to have my best friend Tessa babysit me, or at least stay on the phone with me until it passed. I often pondered how much time it would take to break away from whoever I was with and jump off the nearest bridge. Each time I'd have this intense drive to kill myself. But, thoughts of not being killed by the fall and rather left disabled plagued me. If I were pondering using pills, I would worry that I would end up a vegetable, which would put even more of a burden on my parents. The thoughts that held me back were the possibility that the attempt would not produce fatal results.

I'd come to find years later, that not only was the impulse to take my life made stronger, while under the influence of prescription drugs, the ideations themselves may have been a direct result of the drugs themselves.

By miracle, I am alive today to tell you that a mentally ill, chemically imbalanced person becomes balanced when given the right chemicals and therefore, he steps back from the ledge.

A chemically stable, but emotionally unstable teenager given the same brain altering drugs becomes chemically imbalanced on top of everything else going on in a growing brain, and therefore, he or she is propelled toward the ledge. It is a biochemical equation; imbalanced, apt to jump, balanced naturally but put into a state of artificial imbalance, apt to jump. The latter is possibly even more dangerous than the former. It all depends upon the strength of the imbalance, whether it be biological or pharmaceutical, the equation doesn't change.

Thank You

Steve: for dropping mad wisdom all the time and putting me onto the greatest records!

SG Y: for seeing me and inspiring me with your genius and kind heart.

C: for being my catalyst and for showing me how real men behave.

AA: for keeping my mind right by reading it and throwing out quotes that are scarily on point.

Grandma: for inspiring me through thick and thin and for always giving me a canvas to paint on without judgement.

Parents: for being there, always. I am so blessed.

Thank you Lee C for writing the only books that grounded me in the beginning of this process.

And to Melissa M for shining your light and in turn allowing me to shine mine. (And T of course.)

And thank you Dr. B for saving my life.

Introduction

I'm still not a fan of the vaulted ceilings of this place: my university's twenty-four hour library. Although I enjoyed and still enjoy the time staring up at this majestic ceiling takes away from doing that thing I came to the library to do, I don't exactly appreciate the ceilings for stretching the procrastination out today.

As I move forward in my life and further from the missing years, it is more and more difficult to go back and excavate things. Today it takes a field trip to get back to where I was in order to wrap things up from a sincere place.

This book is the last of three books that delve into the trying environment our country has cultivated. The first two books of the series were heavily steeped in doctor's visits and prescriptions drugs. This last book is a bit different.

Welcome to the last book of The Finding Kali Trilogy, *Finding Kali*. Books 1 & 2, *Losing Kali* and *Missing Kali*, dove into the experiences of falling headfirst into the pharmaceutical industry after a faulty diagnosis of bipolar disorder made in response to my negative reaction to a new prescription of Prozac. The journey of psychotropic drugs began in step with my journey into high school.

Book 2, *Missing Kali*, follows me through ever-shifting prescription drugs, a handful of new doctors, their new diagnoses, and the coinciding

ER visits, some due to long-term effects of drugs stopped in *Losing Kali*, others due to adverse reactions of the new drugs I was given. *Missing Kali* explores new medications for the brand new disorders and syndromes brought to life by new doctors and therapists and their coinciding traumas while I was studying to receive my bachelor's degree at my dream school in less than four years.

Finding Kali follows me after graduation from university and into the world of a bigger pond and more responsibility. Book three, *Finding Kali,* takes me out of the hills that surround my college campus, even out of the country, then up to where the movie stars live and finally into the valley where the recording studios and up-and-coming recording artists thrive.

Something comes out of left field for Kali in this book and it turns the world right onto its head. An unexpected shift of mind, leads to magic far beyond what she had ever imagined.

Nothing was the same.

Finding Kali is like the end of the circle that never ends. It will provide little closure, because these books are about life and therefore, mimic it. This is the last book of the Finding Kali Trilogy, but I hope it is the beginning of a movement toward greater compassion toward one another, courage to tell our stories and passion to hold our flames high as we battle forward into an age just as threatening and just as magical as those we read about in our history books. I hope this marks the beginning of a movement towards justice and the uproar of people like me telling their story, unafraid of the critics and unabashed about the shame they feel.

If you have read the first two books of the series, you will find this book to be very different. I criticized this about myself for a while but always found peace in the fact that it was right, even though it wasn't the same.

Because life is not always so congruent, and because patterns create habitual thinking, and I want to inspire bigger thinking.

I left my original writings, journey scribblings and poetry, in the way I left them, so as to illustrate and preserve my mental state at the time.

I say again, after *Finding Kali*, nothing was the same.

Author's Note <small>[DISCLAIMER: same note as Books 1 & 2)</small>

In the process of writing this third book of three in the Finding Kali Trilogy, I dug into every place I could imagine.

I compiled the journals I had meticulously kept since the invention of the gel pen. I retrieved hard copies of all of my medical records from more than a dozen different sources: doctors, therapists, hospitals, and all the different departments of medicine at the university I attended.

I scoured emails, class assignments from middle school all the way up until my last classes before receiving my B.A. and the scribblings in the margins of my notes from engineering school after that.

I searched obsessively through old social media outlets, not only to find specific dates but to reread painful conversations and find the facts amongst all the feelings. The Facebook messages were some of the worst. I'd since deactivated that account. In reactivating it, I was able to look with a microscope at the random pilings of memories and mishaps.

I typed out each and every one of the journal entries and transcribed the medical records, keepsakes, and notes written by lovers, letters from Grandma, birthday cards, everything. I needed everything I could find, no matter how painful, so that I could to place myself exactly where I had been when things occurred.

I crafted timeline after timeline, linking the medical records and notes, cross-referencing the social media conversations, photographs, and even essays written in class to coinciding events in my life.

I sorted the array of memories in piles by year, then meticulously by month and then even by day in some cases. I had to see things right next to one another, in physical form, to believe that these events happened the way that they did. I couldn't second guess cold hard facts.

For the last couple of books, especially, I retraced my steps back to the actual locations where certain events took place. Sometimes this happened by accident, like today, when I drove past the now redone brick wall I demolished when I first moved to Los Angeles, after applying for a job at that same place under the influence of Lexapro. Other times, I intentionally took a trip into the same places where my life had changed. And it took my breath away more times than I could count.

"It's okay," I would repeat to myself, transported emotionally back to the space in time that held the pain. Sometimes I got lost in the psychological trip of everything. I found myself experiencing the intense depression I used to feel, desperate to grasp on to something that wasn't shifting out from under me. It would take a full night's sleep to remember the power of shifting mindsets and the fact that we create our own realities.

Some memories came as flashbacks at places I frequent now and associate with a completely different life. The places themselves haven't changed at all, yet I hardly recognized them. I get whiplashed with the old emotions and events that transpired there.

I struggled with anger I felt toward a broken system. But also anger with myself for not doing this sooner or not realizing my own worth and getting out of situations before the exit disappeared altogether. And I spent some days mad at others and at the ways we treat each other so differently on this planet even although we are all made up of the same matter.

Having placed pieces of a sometimes intentionally forgotten puzzle back in order, I held my breath and questioned family members to get a full perspective. These were not fun conversations.

I am very auditory and often remember events solely from words exchanged. I crafted dialogue from what I remembered.

Certain people are excluded from the final book to ensure that I portray only the essential characters in getting this message across to you, the reader.

All names of individuals involved (including doctors) have been changed to protect their privacy. At certain times, specific attributes and locations have been changed to preserve the integrity of the individuals and their families.

My goal for this book has nothing to do with pointing fingers at certain people. That will do no good in this situation. My goal is to shed light on an issue that is plaguing us all. We are all in this together, and as one we need to come together and fix this.

I did many hours of research on the effects of pharmaceuticals on our population, pulling from posts on discussion boards as well as articles in medical journals, medical websites, news broadcasts and even the local newspaper.

I did not include these articles in this book in order to preserve the anonymity of the people involved. By directly injecting these stories, I felt it would be overstepping my bounds into a territory that I do not need to cross to tell my story.

Lastly, the Internet searches I performed to locate some of the uniquely corrupt individuals I encountered, brought about an array of incredibly scary results.

However, with much thought, I decided that these, some of whom were even convicted criminals, deserve the right to privacy, and so I held fast to the notion that this is not a book to "out" specific parties, but rather to shed light on a terrible epidemic.

What I can say is that several doctors, as well as people and situations on this harrowing journey, have not only been brought to the of the attention of the general public, but to justice. And some of the large-scale problems I encountered have recently been the topics of news specials and in a few cases, sections of late-night comedy shows.

In order to see the beauty in something, you must stand at a distance and see it from a new angle before returning, whether that takes moments or years.

To fully immerse yourself in a message, you must let it reveal itself in its own time. If you are unable to pull yourself away, unable to hold something loosely, you will never be able to embrace it appropriately and therefore you do not deserve its beauty. You do not recognize the work for what it is, but rather what you see in it. You are only then appreciating yourself: your perception.

If you can't let go and watch something flourish without you, you do not belong in its airspace. Once you detach, you will finally decipher the things you thought were so simple. You might unlock meanings that, until now, remained hidden from you, or new pathways that can now be treasured. You discover new reasons for being a part of this person or this message's life.

The ability to watch a piece of art draw the attention of others, to stimulate a reaction in another's mind and activate some latent memory crucial for this new person's step forward in life, that is brilliance.

In this spirit, I'm stepping back and letting go in the hope that I can save someone else from going through what I went through.

So, here it is.

Namaste.

Kali Rae

Here's to the Brave Ones, the Light Workers, the Warriors...

"It is not the critic who counts; not the man who points out how the strong man stumbles, or where the doer of deeds could have done them better. The credit belongs to the man who is actually in the arena, whose face is marred by dust and sweat and blood; who strives valiantly; who errs, who comes short again and again, because there is no effort without error and shortcoming; but who does actually strive to do the deeds; who knows great enthusiasms, the great devotions; who spends himself in a worthy cause; who at the best knows in the end the triumph of high achievement, and who at the worst, if he fails, at least fails while daring greatly, so that his place shall never be with those cold and timid souls who neither know victory nor defeat" Theodore Roosevelt. *

---

* [Excerpt from the speech "Citizenship In A Republic" delivered at the Sorbonne in Paris, France, on 23 April, 1910].

Abbreviations and Terms

A/P	assessment/plan
Add	additional notes from the doctor or nurse to add to my file
AED	antiepileptic drug
AMA	against medical advice
Asx	asymptomatic
BID	twice a day
BMI	body mass index
c/o	complaints of
CT	or CAT scan, an x-ray scan of your insides
d/c	discontinue
DP	depersonalization, derealization disorder
Dx	diagnosis
ER	emergency room
Etoh	alcohol

F/U	follow up
GAD	generalized anxiety disorder
GP	general practitioner
Hashimotos	an autoimmune disorder where the body attacks the thyroid gland
Hx	history
IC	interstitial cystitis
MD	medical doctor
Mg	milligrams
MRI	magnetic resonance imaging, takes pictures of the insides of your body
MRSA	methicillin-resistant staphylococcus aureus
MVA	motor vehicle accident
N/V	nausea and vomiting
O	"objective" doctor findings and/or results to tests done in the office
PCP	primary care physician
Po	by mouth
Prn	use when necessary, from the Latin phrase, pro re nata, meaning, "as the circumstance arises"
R/sd	rescheduled
Rr	relative risk
Rx	prescription
S	"subjective" information from the patient's perspective
SA	suicide attempts
SI	suicidal ideation
SS	serotonin syndrome
SSRI	selective serotonin reuptake inhibitor
Synthroid	medicine I take for Hashimotos
UTI	urinary tract infection, misdiagnosis, in my case, of kidney stones

VM	voicemail
W	weight
WHNP	women's health nurse practitioner

List Of Doctors

Dr. Aldo, DPT	chiropractor
Dr. Braun, PhD	psychologist at the university's counseling center.
Dr. Calvin, MD	psychiatrist at the university
Dr. Daus, MD	urgent care physician, also Beau's dad.
Dr. Douglas, MD	my general practitioner at the university
Dr. Fiaschetti, MD	long-distance, long-term psychiatrist, referred by Dr. Sandy after Dr. Morano has a mental break and nearly kills me with meds, located on the coast, closer to Newport than LA.
Dr. Jane, MD	my original general practitioner and the mother of Dr. Scott
Dr. Jensen, MD	psychiatrist who gives me Prozac in tenth-grade, ups the dose and leaves the country
Dr. Kate, MFT	psychologist referred by Dr. Braun, works at BHI on campus (behavioral health institute)
Dr. Morano, MD	previous psychiatrist who was tased in his back yard, a general practitioner acting as a psychiatrist

Dr. Nguyen, MD radiologist

Dr. Olivera, MD neurologist

Dr. Roberts, MD urgent care physician in Newport

Dr. Sandy, PhD beloved psychologist I am linked up with after Portofino rehab stay in high school

Dr. Scott, MD long-term general practitioner in Newport, also the son of Dr. Jane, primary care physician who labeled me bipolar after my reaction to Prozac in high school, oversaw care while I was at university

Dr. Thompson, MD first psychiatrist I ever visited, in fourth grade because of my sister getting drunk in Palm Springs

Dr. Whittman, PhD first psychologist I ever visited, tricked me and sent me to rehab for an eating disorder, reason for my trust issues around therapists

1 Days in the East

The Cast Party

My apartment's carpets even smell new. My parents helped me move in this past weekend. Everything was incredibly tame. I even had the internet hooked up by the early afternoon.

The large window facing opposite the door was a top selling point, and I smile at my choice as the August sunlight streams into my apartment expanding it even further as I pull on the ball-chain to bring the sunlight onto my bed.

This apartment is a lot bigger and a lot more "traditional." So I can put away all of my things, with extra room in the upper kitchen cabinets. It is unheard of to have this kind of space after getting used to a bed that can be pushed up against the wall during the day to work on projects, or to make space for the pile of beads I am organizing or creating from.

The day before moving in I tell Brent that I need space. I allow him to come over to collect his Red Stripe t-shirt but tell him he shouldn't come back. I lie when I say that I am in love with my ex. JJ. It is easier to get away that way.

My empathy toward Brent turned to irritation pretty shortly after he came over acting like a tweaker. Brent is not the person I met anymore, and he is scaring me. It also pisses me off that he tries to pass as the cordial guy I met outside of my Shakespeare class on the vivid green grass of a California July on campus.

"You have to meet my friend Andriy!" Julian says excitedly, "He's in the music industry too, you'd love him. Come to the cast party. We'll bring him."

This comment streaks across my memory as I debate going to the party or not. I respond to Julian's text, agreeing to accompany him and his friend, Victor, to the cast party.

Me: Yeah. I'd love to come!

That night at the Brendon, Julian had played the role of the 'bartender.' We spent hours laughing as he fake-poured my drink, over and over and over and over again. Victor sat directly to my left at the bar. And depending on the take he would join in, fake-spilling on me, or just plain hitting on me.

It is an impressive crew within the dozens of other actors on set. The extras are friends of the director. And they are amusing.

I clip-clop on the summer night's pavement and go from new-apartment smell into new-car smell, as I pull my dress down, trying to navigate my black bootie-heals into the back seat of Julian's blacked-out BMW.

"Nice car!" I say as I pull my dress down, navigating the entrance so that I don't flash everyone.

"Thank you," Julian says.

"What's up, girl!" Victor turns around in the passenger seat to give me a fist-bump, which I turn into an awkward hand-grab, like a Rock, Paper, Scissors, game. I'm not skilled at that greeting, ever.

We arrive at Julian's Beverly Hills home. It is the house where Julian grew up. The sun is just about completely gone behind the black of the summer night. A tall boy in dark denim, burgundy leather shoes and a cardigan walks up the tile steps onto the porch of the adobe-style home.

Okay, he's super cute. I hope this is the house.

"Speaking of the devil! Andriy!" Victor catcalls to the tall boy.

"That's the Canadian," Julian says, catching my eyes in the rearview mirror.

"Canadian? For real?" I ask.

Julian laughs and says, "Yes, Kali. Andriy's really Canadian…" Julian teases me by exaggerating the "'really'" in his answer, "why?"

"Oh! I don't know," I say.

A Rescue Attempt

I have three bottles of Pink Zinfandel lined up by the entrance to 'The Nook.' 'The Nook' is the name I gave the small, under the stairs-like area within my walk-in closet on Beverly. Ever since meeting JJ and sleeping in the attic-like space of Sunset/Bronson studios, I obsessed over finding small places to sleep. It brought me back to my childhood.

The Nook is located within the large walk-in closet in the apartment I moved into after my mom stepped in regarding Brent and the ridiculous situation at the second Carmelina apartment. Never again will she trust my decision in finding apartments.

This new-age Nook is perfect. It is the reason I decided on this place. It is big enough to fit a full sleeping bag. The Nook is tucked away enough to feel completely isolated from the rest of the apartment, but also, the rest of the world. The walk-in closet door securely shuts and the step down into The Nook provides extra superficial safety.

No overly emotional song lyrics will escape The Nook and entertain the passing neighbors. It gives me a space to be completely open and alone.

I stay up all night in there: writing, crying and drinking.

Within a couple of weeks, and with Christina's help, I begin to make the Nook's walls a mural, quoting my favorite musicians, painting their lyrics on the walls. Christina joins in decorating the walls of the Nook with her art.

She draws and paints in there like it is her private canvas. It is a beautiful mix of fragments of songs and wandering line paintings. It is fun to trace

Christina's lines around to find they make faces: people amongst the lyrics strewn about.

Tonight, I bring my computer, my journal and re-rent *Blue Valentine*. I cry within the confines of that blank space. It isn't broken in just yet. I turn the movie on silent and play "Wicked Games" on repeat; a song that the Canadian boy from that cast party gave me, and I cry more. I cry until I can't see the page I am writing on.

I finish the first bottle, throw it out into the walkway of the walk-in closet, hoping it shatters dramatically, but it disappoints, bouncing into Stella's toy basket instead.

Stella, who's been hanging in the Nook with me, perks up a little. I recognize how pitiful I am when I realize that Stella is witnessing this breakdown. I shuffle into the kitchen, grab a bottle-opener, and the antibiotic prescribed for the millionth kidney infection am currently battling.

I think back to the way JJ showed up in the new apartment with a bag of groceries but didn't stay. I thought of the way his gesture mocked the atmosphere of what I thought was a much more mature apartment. His condescending presence made everything seem childish. And I wanted him to stay. He still hadn't forgiven me for the comment I made about seeing ghosts, or for making him sleep on the mess of clothes from the solo move-in because HE didn't show up. But anyway, I still wanted him to stay that night. I wanted to be wanted by somebody.

I shuffle back into the closet and duck under the low hanging entrance and crawl under the comforter.

"I am about to be very drunk, Stella," I say and take a swig.

Fuck it.

Stella looks worried.

"Love you, Boo!" I coax.

I un-mute my new favorite film and start working on a new bottle of wine.

A few minutes in, a text comes through. It's from that Canadian music guy, Andriy:

Andriy: Yo, I'm with Victor, Julian and Jamie, come out with us, I'm right next to your place.

I'm amazed that someone cares about me and more amazed that I was amazed by that fact. I sob more, too tired to filter my response.

Me: I'm a mess, in a nook, drinking wine, thanks for the song.

I don't get a response. I didn't think I would. I wouldn't respond to that. I am too sad to care anymore that I may have embarrassed myself to someone I don't know.

Andriy: Kali turn off "Wicked Games" please. You are abusing it. Also, put clothes on, we will be there in 10. P.S you helped me the other night. Now it's my turn.

The Hearing

My palms are sweaty as I press them together. I button and rebutton the top button of my black sweater.

"You ready, sweetie?" my father asks.

"Yeah, just nervous," I say.

I speak quietly as if responding to a reading of the Miranda Rights. I uncross my legs and cross my feet instead. The flats I'm wearing are sticky. My toes slip past one another.

"Ms. Wheeler? Officer Ernst is ready for you," a pencil-skirted woman says.

"Okay, great. Thanks!" I blurt out. I'm a little too excited as I carefully stand up and flatten my skirt back down. I walk towards the door and my dad grabs my left shoulder.

"Breathe," he says.

I nod.

We are led into a small room. There are certificates on the wall and a woman behind a large wood desk. A tape recorder is set up alongside a couple piles of paper. There are two chairs on our side.

"Hello! How are you two this morning?" the officer says.

"I'm good; how are you?" I reply, strangely confident in relation to my first encounter with her assistant.

"Good, good." My father pauses for a moment. "Well, ready to get this all resolved." His attorney-bred composure shines like always.

"Well, that's exactly what we are here to do. Please take a seat," the officer responds.

The wood legs of the chair don't make it easy to pull the chair across the carpet and slip in. I fumble a bit awkwardly to slip into the minimal space allowed between the chair and desk. I don't want to seem uptight by fumbling anymore with the heavy chair.

"I need to let you know that we will be recording this hearing. This is the proceeding for the reinstatement or revocation of your Class B License, suspended on the morning of April the 20th after a collision with two vehicles in which you experienced a lapse of consciousness. If you agree to the terms of this hearing repeat after me; I, then state your name, am aware that the hearing will be recorded," the officer says.

"I, Kali Rae Wheeler…" I repeat.

The hearing begins, not unlike I had planned, the honest background information I gave my neurologist becomes the talking point for the license revocation and suspension.

I gave this information to the neurologist, Dr. Olivera, in his cold office on the other side of town, in hopes that he would understand more about me holistically and therefore be able to help me figure out what had happened that afternoon after my mammoth trip. I didn't think it would be turned against me as a case for my license suspension. The doctor asked me if I ever "engage" in any drinking. And, not thinking it had to do with my license, I explained that I had been in the program and that when I drink, I black out, which is why I don't like to drink.

I respond without a filter to Dr. Olivera because that's how my mind works. I am not a schemer. I don't think twice about it.

The truth is, if I weren't under the influence of personality-affecting medication, I probably would have been savvy enough to mark the box "no," next to alcohol use on Dr. Olivera's stupid form. Since I wasn't twenty-one at the time, and I guess that is just what you do when asked questions on questionnaires; if it doesn't pertain to the exact symptom you are at the doctor to sort out, you mark "no." Too much information can harm you.

The conversation regarding alcohol continued with Dr. Olivera because of my blatant admission of having a "problem." He reacted as if he understood the disease and like he, himself, was also part of the program. Unable to conceal my cellular recognition of him, I continued to reveal my background. His caring, blue eyes enthralled me and unraveled my deepest secrets while he continued to assure me of his understanding and acknowledgment of it all.

He affirmed me with things like:

"You're so young. You must have an old soul to have already discovered that this is an issue for you." And his comment to me upon leaving: "You're a wise girl. Kali, stay sober. You are going to do great things."

The whole experience was uplifting, actually, and all of the tests he ran were negative.

I regarded this information as helpful guidance, without a clue that he would decide, without any other reasoning, note that alcohol has been a problem in my past and that he has advised me to stay sober.

'Excuuuuse me sir, that was told to you in confidence … and now I just look like a drunk who crashed, thanks.

Blue Heights: Intro to New Heights

I take MDMA for the first time when it is carefully purchased by my physicist/genius-neighbor Felix. Felix is Christina's ex-boyfriend. He is also the guy who saves me from myself by engaging me in philosophical conversations over a Camel Crush at four a.m., both of us aware and accepting of our current states of insanity. The guilt I feel being a little reckless vanishes. It is okay to be a little bit bad.

I learn to appreciate the feeling of the night escaping us; the sun always rises too soon for us to finish what we planned to finish that night.

Because we chose to procrastinate doing our assignment until the very last night, it gives us both momentum and in turn, inertia, to press on.

It is exciting to be a bit crazed with Felix. Because it is our decision.

It is our decision to procrastinate all night long, meet up, talk at first about the projects we are working on, and then admit the holes we wander down in the process of finishing. In my case, the course diverts from the essay on the Victorian era into researching the theories behind sacred geometry. Meanwhile, Felix is neglecting to study for his molecular bio exam, and instead, is trying to calculate the density of dark matter.

The first time I take MDMA I don't feel anything.

The next time I take it. I come alive. I feel, for the first time ever, comfortable, happy to be here and able to accept things in my past. I mostly find myself in a place of non-judgment, not separating the past "wrongs" from the future "rights" I am able to simply live and to take a huge sigh of relief.

I smile.

And I mean it.

The magic rests in the acceptance that we are all still searching for something to bring us to life.

Felix accompanies Andriy and me on my first truly exceptional night. He provides the Molly, supposedly "pure ecstasy." It is the expensive kind, free of contaminants. It is an event just to get the pills that at first do nothing for me. And then all at once, they do EVERYTHING for me.

Bring the 7-0-7 Out

My new favorite soundtrack blares over the speakers in the Range Rover as I rediscover Los Angeles from its roots to its tips with my tour guide, a Canadian transplant, Andriy, and a companion, Felix. Felix is so high on E that when I turn around to show him the feeling of "AHHHHHH!! This is so coooooool!" he is literally in a ball, inside his sweatshirt, smiling so wide I swear I could feel it in the front seat.

He looks adorable; a childhood innocence radiates through him like he is opening presents on Christmas morning: a pure happiness haze.

I think the happiness I am feeling may have also projected onto Felix a bit too. We are all enamored with life.

My favorite alternative R&B song makes my stomach jump into my throat as I record the drive on my phone. Streetlights pass like stars in my own private galaxy. The familiar bassline jolts my seat into overdrive. Abel Tesfaye croons as the beat drops out, switching the song into overdrive. I moan to no one in particular, "I am so in love."

Andriy reaches over to grasp the top of my knee. He squeezes it hard and looks at me with his 'love you like crazy' look from the film *Blue Valentine*. Andriy loved the part of that film where the lead character, Ryan Gosling, scrunches up his face and says, "Love you like CRAAAZY!" to his four-year-old daughter.

We are heading to Blue Heights first, an overlook of the entire city of Los Angeles that will soon become my favorite place on the planet.

My heart leaps as I get out of the car, in awe of the round, almost malleable space concept we find ourselves in atop this mountain that overlooks all of the sparkling lights of my city. I am awake, attentive, yet so able to be grateful and appreciative of the moment. I have no barriers. Not one part of my mind stops me when I am feeling great to say:

"Whoa, wait up there Kali. Something bad's going to happen now. We aren't allowed to feel this good."

I got rid of all that.

I am set free. Above the city tonight, staring down on all the places I traversed in the past years. I feel like I am flying into the center of it all.

For the first time since everything started way back in middle school, I can breathe again. The twinkling lights of the city look docile and wise. A familiar and foreign feeling washes over me as Andriy squeezes my hand.

Everything is available to me. The city is like a younger sibling who needs direction. A comfortable feeling washes over me with even more intensity: a feeling of being in love with being alive in this moment and intrinsically connected to the people I love. This love is universal. There are no boundaries or time constraints or "too-earlys." I can do anything and I always could. All of the interest in the law of attraction and things from out of this world, a oneness that connects the globe, it is all real. (See Appendix J).

Los Angeles and its bright lights nearly blinded me, but they didn't and now I rise stronger and more invigorated than ever before.

It's time.

"You like it?" Andriy asks.

His eyes are sparkling and his pupils are so big he looks like a Keen painting in the best way.

"I'm in love with it!" I say.

Before I can stop smiling from the question, Andriy grabs my hand, squeezes it tightly and stands up. As a gentleman would, he helps me up and pulls me to him for one last glance before shouting to Felix, who has been roaming somewhere. I watch him bound toward us, arms pulled into his hoodie like a kid, his sandy blonde hair poofing out of the gray Sailing Team hoodie. He is smiling wide and bringing good vibes to the couple walking up the path from the parking lot in the big black night.

"There's somewhere else I need to take you," Andriy says. "Felix have you been to the caves?"

"Aw, man! In Malibu? Yes but that's the best plan, " Felix says.

"What caves?" I ask.

"Come on!" Andriy playfully grabs me to head back to the car. It's a good thing he did or I would have stayed on the dirt path all night. I was in ecstasy, literally. And I was so ready to fall into the center of the love I was feeling for Andriy, for myself, for Felix, for Los Angeles, for the universe. I was blissed out.

The lights of the streetlamps fly past like one of those postcards of a rainy day. I am perfectly stable without having to keep still. I am weaving in the passenger seat, grinding to another one of my new favorite songs. Andriy is the best at cultivating mixtapes.

Frank Ocean's debut hit single hits just the right chord at just the right time.

Soon we are miles up the coast in Malibu.

I immediately take off my UGG boots and sprint from the parking lot into the cool sand of the dark beach, plunging my feet in and feeling the cold wind whip against my face. I make it all the way to the water.

The boys are standing on the shore.

"Come on!" I shout to the two of them but they can't hear me and wave instead.

AWWW.

I dip my toes in and run back to them after playing catch me if you can with the tide. The stars are like pinpoints in a piece of paper backlit in a dark room.

I lose sight of the boys for a minute, staring up the beach in the opposite direction. The emptiness is interesting, but I want to be around Andriy and Felix.

I find them wandering into a nearby cave, Felix is holding my UGGs.

My heart flutters again.

"Thank you!" I say without filtering my excitement. I would have totally lost those and they're my favorite boots.

"Of course," Felix smiles.

"Have you been in the caves?" Andriy asks?

"No, but it's kind of sketchy at night, right?" I say, "Like people having sex, sketchy."

"Let's build a sandcastle instead," Felix offers.

"I'm so down!"

I decide to grab life by the horns that summer; to write embarrassing love letters, to cut out photos of the two of us, within the two weeks of our meeting. I want to be best friends and partners in exploration, and I want Felix to come too! And Christina!

I accept that the idea of love is not one that requires anything in return, not even the affection from the other. It transcends all that and places you above anything that could ever steal it away from you. It just is what it is when it is, where it is, but there is no, why it is.

Confirming the Ticket

I spend hours on the phone with my mother asking her if I should book the ticket or not.

"I just met him. His friends are nice. So he's not a serial killer. I don't think," I say into the phone.

"Kali, you can't just go to Canada!" my mom says, nearly shouting.

"That's the thing. I totally can. And I will," I say.

That's it; I'm going.

That is the final time I try and prove my reasoning to her. There is no sound reasoning for this trip, and that is the point.

But I hang up the phone, just to call right back. It is a sick game that I do not mean to play. I am asking for approval for something she does not approve. It is a lose-lose situation.

I text Christina, but I don't expect a text back. She isn't good at things like texting.

> *Me: What if I don't have a place to stay? Like what if he just says he wants me to come, but he doesn't?*
>
> *Christina: Fuck it, man, don't listen to anyone, do what you want. Book the flight. Live a little!*

I watch the ellipses bounce up and down:

> *Christina: Put clothes on. I'm coming over*

"CONFIRM BOOKING?" I look intently at the square yellow button, wondering why it was necessary for the airline to place a question mark in there. It's not like we aren't questioning the decision to fly away from wherever we are. I race through my thoughts once more, just for old time's sake. A wave of adrenaline rushes through me. I'm gone.

Click.

Did I do it?

I wait for the confirmation page to load, unsure if I pressed the button. The confirmation headline centers itself on the webpage: "BOOKING CONFIRMED."

I did it!

Yes

Yes

YES!

I'm going to TORONTO! 6 SIDE† WAH?!

It is at the moment I decide to say "fuck it" that the real magic begins. It is at the time that I throw out all of my ideas about shoulds and be reckless, this time in a vulnerable way, that things take flight.

I am used to being reckless within my zone of comfort. As the youngest, I can get myself into trouble and know that I will make it out. I have the support of my older brother and my parents to play the padding on the walls of my self-imposed cell of insanity. Kayla is there to test me in that room. She is there to throw the curve-balls, to ask me twice, to ridicule me because I need to learn how to fight back. I do not learn how to fight back until I learn how to let go. Toronto is the first time I decide to let go of all of the things I know to do when I don't know what to do.

---

† I am a bit obsessed with Toronto, and a bit entranced by the music coming out of the area at the time. The 6, or 6ix, is a nickname for Toronto that isn't new, but it recently gained popularity when the music industry started blowing up with stars from Toronto.

Near-Death Preludes

I have felt the feeling of death twice. Both times, I prayed for it: so that I would not be afraid of death anymore. And both times, a sense of complete and utter bodilessness and comfort surround me: a sense of returning home. There is no pain or suffering, just quiet realization.

The first near-death illusion/vision comes in a dream: death via drowning. I watch myself fall through the water, like a movie, but I feel the character's emotions because I am the character drowning. The feeling is all-immersive. It is warm—not hot—just comfortable.

Every ache in my body that, even at a young age, reminds you that you're human, falls away. I am slowly falling deeper and deeper below the water's surface. It is daytime because the rays of the sun penetrate the top section of water as I fall farther away from them. There isn't any fear of the darker water below because it is unnecessary. I am focused on my quiet, motionless freefalling through the sunlit ocean water. I watch the particles of miniature creatures and things dance in the beams of light through the water, too small for the human eye to decipher. My hair fans out around me, mermaid-like. I am leaving now.

Before I pass into the darker water below, I wake up.

Never once do I see anything but light: the sun gleams through the water above as I fall without a fight, slowly.

The second dream occurs after September 11, 2001. I am in middle school. With the threat of the Middle East on every news channel and sprawled across every magazine and newspaper headline, I guess it was only normal to fear there would be an attack.

The dream places me in my high school locker room. There is a loud, ear-ringing blast, and then a comedic, caricature "POW!" logo flashes across my mind: red, yellow, and orange zigzags frame it.

I jump under one of the locker room benches, and a familiar warmth floods my body. This time the yellow haloed white light encompasses my surroundings. The light comes in from all directions and swallows the locker room. I am not earthbound anymore. It happens instantly. The bright yellow-lined, white light consumes the locker room. It is like a very much cooler version of what scientific pictures of the sun look like, but instead of orange flames coming from the center the ball of white light is surrounded by a corona of yellow haze. This time, it feels that my surroundings on Earth have been obliterated and instead of witnessing an earthbound situation I am transported through time and space into the very center of the light.

Once again, I acknowledge the overwhelming joyful feeling of being home again. I am peaceful, protected, and warm. Things are not needing to be solved or climbed out of; I am where I am supposed to be, and this is the time I will return home.

I find the distinct feeling, again, of bodilessness. I don't have a body or not have a body. I am concentrated, but not all in the same space at the same time. It is an all-seeing, all-feeling presence, which is hard to explain in a linear fashion. The realm I am in made these experiences one in the same: I simply am. I feel space, not tangibly, but energetically. I have a presence that is now overseeing the experience of human life.

The love surrounding me envelopes me in a calm ecstasy. It's not connected to a single entity, but rather is all around me.

I wake up astounded by the beautiful calm this dream brings. It reinvigorates the idea that I am part of a bigger puzzle.

I have also been in the in-between. I don't exactly call it a near-death experience because it wasn't my time yet. It could be called a hiccup: a hiccup in my personal matrix. And whoever is up there wasn't going to let me leave Earth yet.

I mistakenly come farther over the edge than I expected. In order to keep from tipping, I experience a vision that reaches past my physical reality and pulls me back into my conscious state. I wake up with a start in a dark bedroom, adrenaline halting the signs of my hangover until a few moments later.

This last and most recent experience is one that I didn't recognize until recently, due to my inability to sort through events and karmic relations with other people while so heavily medicated.

August 15, 2011

Just keep drinking, sweetie, drink more love, drink until you can't see…
XO Kali Rae
(See Appendix I, K.)

August 16, 2011

And I can't even write without returning
to the eyes that cut me so deep
Baby you ain't seen nothing yet
You will be my muse
As I walk through this life
Building an empire that no one could break

If I could see you
This darkness would turn to light

I'd rather watch you leave
And deal with my pain of missing those beautiful eyes
Than sit here wondering why I let you go

I don't know if you're the one
And I don't know if things will ever
Pan out like they should

All I want
And all I need
Is oxygen to sustain me
And re-assurance that the candle that burns alongside my chaos and
random scribblings
Did not burn in vain

Because Baby I do not care to share
I do not bock anymore
I am ready to fall
If you'd like to fall with me
I'd catch you
Distance doesn't separate
Something that resonates so deeply within me
If it does
I do not care
I know I'll cry watching you leave
And it's not me to feel this way
Neither is it me to let you see this
I don't know what love is
But I thank you for showing me it's possible
Do this for me...

Simply remember me
Because what I need from you is nothing more than the reassurance that
this was something special

You have actually given me something I've never felt before
And I wouldn't compromise my life for something that could be fantasy
But I think that I'm falling in love with you
And don't think you won't be getting letters
Thank you for giving me something I've never had
And no, I didn't know I was beautiful
Until you said so

Sometimes I can't breathe
Listening to a rhythm that I can't even try to complete
One more time
Give me one more
One more rhyme
Cuz I…
I can't even try to reconcile
This one
This time
One time
Where leaving messages simply won't suffice
I lost you
The day I lost that in my eye
My eye
I and I
Can't even try
I want this but try not to take this
Take it, place it up and away
For you I found a place to hide
My broken frame
Cuz I…

Give one more laugh
I'll give one more cry
Maybe
Baby
When you're
I can't take take away the
Words you've written in my songs
Wait for me
Wait

Give it back
Give

Because standing here next to you
It's like I can't even say
All the things I know you've wanted to as well
When I stop and stare
It's there
It's there
It's here

Reaching Out, The Hallway: August 29, 2011

I'm wearing a Christina custom-designed dress and a gun necklace that I crafted from the little metal gun charm that Brent gave me. The dress is left over from one of Christina's fabric projects. I stick on Christina's black bowler hat just for kicks, the one with the speckled feather sticking out of the side. I should be packing for my trip to Toronto, but instead, I am going with Christina to a party across the street. I promised her I would check it out.

Once at the stuffy apartment across the street from my Beverly Street apartment, I drink whiskey, beer, and whatever else the boys pour for me. The guys on the balcony are smoking weed and being social butterflies I manage to get talking to the boys who brought it. They offer it to me.

I spend the first hour tossing back the ever-changing and ever-replenishing liquid in my red Solo cup while taking hits from the little pipe the boys load and reload with abandon.

The next thing I remember is being on the couch. My face leaning into my right palm, elbow on the right arm of the chair, Christina walks over and asks me if I am okay.

I want to speak, but all I can get out are these huffs of air and quiet squeaking/whining sounds. My arm gives way, and my head bobs off my palm, slumping me over to the side. The iron curtains of my eyelids drop over my eyes and everything goes black.

I am fully conscious, but my brain is not listening to what I am telling it. I cannot open my eyes, and I cannot feel any part of my body.

Christina calls to me again, and she is far away this time. It seems like she is in a different reality, a different part of space-time.

"Kali! Kali! Please get up for me."

I manage to peek out of the bottom of my heavy eyelids and see only an orange blur for a second before the curtain falls again. It's quick and cumbersome. I know I'm not coming out of this. I pray to be spared, just this last time.

Christina's arms wrap under my armpits and lock behind my back as she begs: "Kali, you need to stand up now. I can't lift you. Stand up for me. Please!" I feel her strength lift me off the sofa and then my toes dragging against the carpet.

Everything feels like lead.

And then, the scene behind my eyelids changes. I am suddenly in a hallway. I don't see myself from above, but rather I have become a new form, not my human self. The tangibility of the hallway is Earth-like, but not of Earth, or at least anything I have seen ever seen before.

The walls are dark, maybe cement, but they look black in the darkness. The ceilings are taller than the width of the hallway. It's foggy or dusty. It isn't completely lit up, but there is a light coming from the right side of the darkish hallway that emanates far past its location. It lights up the otherwise dark hall in that the particle of dust shimmers as the fronds of light pass through the air.

It creates the effect that comes about when you look over the ocean at sunset after a rainstorm: when the clouds open up, and the light from the hidden sun illuminates the sky like beams into the heaven.

It's a lot less dramatic in scope, and the source of the light is not uncomfortably bright. I squint a bit and then relax. I walk forward, toward the light, as I had told my grandfather to do several years before he passed.

It doesn't seem like a long distance to walk until I've begun. I never quite caught up to the source of the light. It turns out to be a little farther than I'd estimated. A disembodied, radiating bluish arm appears from the right side above me.

"It's not time yet. Let's go," voice says politely but sternly.

I immediately recognize it as a guide of mine. I grab the arm.

The light gets farther away as we touch. I hesitate, and the grip loosens, the light gets closer.

Just for a moment, I feel his grasp lessen until the disembodied hand squeezes mine a little harder and reinforces: "Let's go!" I feel him tug me in the opposite direction of the light. "Not now, Kali. We've got things to do."

I wake up in a pitch-black room. Christina is lying next to me. She gasps and swings her hand across my chest onto my heart with a thud.

She looks like she's been up for days.

I gather information slowly. I don't have any idea of time, but my moment of insight lasted over four excruciating hours, Christina reports: FOUR hours out-cold.

I pull myself together relatively quickly. We walk home to my apartment across the street from the party. Christina is stunned that I'm conscious. She's in a zombie-like state, freaked-out because she'd fallen asleep, drunk in her efforts to get me to the hospital. I'm stunned by what I've just seen and the feeling of extreme gratitude and awe. I'm high on life.

I call Andriy later to tell him that I saw him in the tunnel: to tell him that he saved me, that he reached his arm out to me and bargained with me to come out of where I was heading. At this time, Andriy is the archetype of my protector. I believe that it is him who holds all of my strength. It was his hands that put me back together that night in August when my pieces were scrambled. He's held me together ever since.

My altered state of mind connects Andriy with all that is good. If I had had my impulses in check that night, I would not have almost died by failing to account for the things I put into my body.

Falling Faster with Big Pharma

And you wonder, okay, how does this have anything to do with Big Pharma? Well, here ya go:

I fall harder and faster than ever before, and I eventually become overwhelmed by what I create. Andriy is an escape from the trivialities and errands of each day. He is an interruption in the redundancy, and since he is so far away, I can melt any idea I have into what he does or says.

I create him and tailor him in my mind to fit what I need, and to make him, literally, God-sent. I make decisions that a logical person would find terrible. We sleep in a park, roll on Ecstasy and drink everything we can get our hands on. We are reckless but careful with one another.

"Let's go!" Andriy says. his pupils are dilated, and his hand feels like a warm, scratchy glove clasping mine to lead me forward into the reality that I have created, have allowed myself to feel. I feel safer than I have felt since I was a child.

We both aren't interested in claiming each other. Our confidence lets an amazing thing bloom. I can love with all of my heart and want nothing in return.

It feels amazing to spend hours working on a card to give to Andriy, not knowing if he will find it weird or overly interested. I love doing it because I love the headspace I create around having Andriy in my life.

It is the process that matters for me. The complete annihilation of the walls I built up so strong is only possible due to the frailty of my emotional state. It is the smoothie of ingredients that allow for this avalanche to gain momentum.

Andriy, and the adventures of finding myself by finding the light I can provide for someone else, cause a tropical storm in my life. It is draining, but so fulfilling. It is love with no boundaries, no remorse and no expectations for reciprocation. I don't care. The simple things mean everything.

The first time I go to Toronto, I happen to arrive the day Andriy is moving out of his apartment. The process of finding a place in Toronto is somewhat similar to the difficulty of finding a place in New York City; you need an agent and everything.

Amidst phone-calls from real estate brokers and possible roommates, I have the genius idea of heading to the local department store to take a nap on one of their extra fluffy beds. We slept at a luxurious hotel the night before, the Royal York, which Andriy so valiantly stepped up and booked in desperation for our situation.

We sleep great in the department store too. It makes people smile, and we are only kicked out after being given a very nice compliment by the store manager.

"You guys are great models for the bedding sets!" the store employee says gleefully.

At this specific time in my life, the medications I swallow ease the prior pain and allow me to feel the marvelous roller coaster. The drugs create the roller coaster. They allow me to have bumpers where there should be hard boundaries.

And Molly heals my depression one evening while I stare up at the clock tower in Nathan Phillips Square. I can finally see the bigger picture.

The months with Andriy in Canada are soaked in audible ecstasy too after Andriy shows me some of my very favorite alternative, hip hop artists. They make it feel like it is okay not to be alright. And don't we all just want to be accepted for who we are now? They are reckless, uninhibited and downright irresponsible in so many ways, but nevertheless, these months were the best months of my life.

The "Fuck It" Magic, Ascending North

The magic of summer gives way to an even greater magic. The magic of learning how to do exactly what you want to do, when you want to do it. The magic of finding the immense power that hides where you'd least expect it. The power of saying "no" because you want to, and say "yes" just because you feel like it.

Being intentionally reckless taught me how to live life. Before that moment, I'd been a victim of my circumstances. But now, I was taking back control and I was taking responsibility. If the trip failed, I'd be okay with that, because *it was mine*.

It was the same freedom and exhilaration, the pure awe that swept through me like the waves that brought me out to sing that explicit rap song with Emma while high on Prozac. Except this time, it was self-made.

I am swept into motion: into a sea of events that won't be perfect. They will hurt, even *a lot* at times. Things will hurt even more than I have hurt up to that point, but it gives me a reason to stay, to push past the obstacles in order to find *this* space we once had. It is a continual race to find a space of rediscovery: the space I found with Andriy driving down sunset listening to "Glass Table Girls" or running around Toronto without a place to stay.

I am liberated. I am the world's muse. I am in rapture. I am entranced by the pure plausibility of changing it all. The tattoo on Andriy's chest emblazons itself on my mind: "It is in your moments of decision that your destiny is shaped."

Things Make Sense: The Jack Layton Memorial

As we come across the tall clock tower, the Canadian National Tower lights up, changing colors, red and purple, then watercolor-like. I run up the steps into the center of what I find out later is Nathan Phillips Square.

I stand in pure exhilaration reading the messages of love transcribed in so many different languages written in chalk on the walls of the square. (See Appendix J.)

"It's a memorial for Jack Layton…He's a politician," Andriy says approaching me from behind but staying far enough away for me to have my moment.

I am speechless. I break away again to stare at the arches spanning the square.

It all makes sense. It all comes together right there. It is all going to be just fine. There is more.

The message I get that night is one that I've cherished ever since. Staring up into the perfect skyline, the clock tower, the CN Tower, and the nearly full moon, this foreign place with such a familiar warmth, the cool air of the evening saving everything in a perfectly crisp breath of brand new.

I am reborn that night.

I didn't choose to be, but life chose me.

A Painful Realization above a New City

Andriy can tell I'm holding back tears as I scrunch up my nose and shake my hair a couple of times. I run my fingers through its scraggly ends. It's a realization I'm having that life is fleeting. As much as I want to relax into it, time passes even if we don't stay aware.

"I want you to keep that key," I say.

Andriy thanks the waitress as she sets down another lychee martini for me, and a whiskey sour for him.

My eyes don't stray. I'm trying to save him in my mind: to capture his essence to take back with me to LA.

I want so desperately to bottle up the feeling of that moment, so freed by the ability to let the small stuff go, and to realize the greatness that the world has to offer us, to save this feeling of freedom and responsibility, to bring it home with me, to continue to cut the chains our minds are so accustomed to fastening around things we want to keep. I want to hold this piece of time, in this foreign place, loosely, so it doesn't break.

I feel like I am playing that sick game "catch the dollar." The game where someone drops a one hundred dollar bill between your hands and your reflexes are too slow to catch it. It inevitably falls through your fingertips, even though it seems like it's right there for us to snatch.

"Want to know something, Kali?"

I am shocked by his candor. He never acts this way. His eyes lock into mine instead of darting to either direction. I take in the awe of the moment; this time he is right there with me.

The sun streams through the glass at Milestones, a restaurant that overlooks the bustling Toronto square below and takes me back to the first night I stumbled into this magic place.

I catch of glimpse of The Bond Place Hotel and get a pang of nostalgia remembering our recovery morning there. The night before, we had to make sure we had bought enough alcohol to last through the night since the liquor stores close early in Canada. (They have lots of rules about when and where you can purchase alcohol in Canada, so you've actually got to plan your getting drunk).

"You want to know the moment I fell in love with you?"

My eyes widen. I try to remember to relax and breathe normally so as not to look completely insane.

"It was when you were in the pub that I made us check out. You were staring at the bookshelf. You had this thing around you, this light; I don't know how to explain it." He takes a sip of the tall golden beer that was just placed in front of him. "And then you laughed at something you were reading. You lit up even more, and then you brought it to me, the book, but you also brought over the light, your light, without even knowing the joy you had given me."

Poems from the Flight Back to Lalaland

[September 3, 2011]

Not Quite Sure Why

The organization of this journal reflects the
disorienting pattern of my life.
Yeah I'm 20.
Clap for me
as I graduate another statistic,
another uneducated university graduate.

I'm not quite sure why
ever.
I'm not quite sure why
I've never.
But today I'm quite sure
that forever,
is something I've learned to cherish.

I used to pray about the process of dying,
and I've recited
over and over
why forever
is just not tangible
nor desired.

But now I see
more than ever before,
that I'm flying Continental
And I've never felt so sure
That forever is such a
beautiful incongruity
when spent under the haven
of a lover's dreaming tree.

If I

If I
Were to disregard the mixture
swirling so elegantly
all into one

If I
Were to forget the beauty
Of playful playmates
Digging together
Digging our tiny hands into
The grainy sand to nowhere
But unintentionally
Anywhere but the sandbox
We were confined in

If I
Were to push away the dirty fingers
Pressing upon my
Delicate skin
And if I
Were to teach the world
Of all the pain it impresses
On itself
Well Maybe
Just maybe the light would
break through and warm
The icicles that inhabit my room.

If there was a way
To turn all the unfit
Moments into clear cut
Pieces of a more important puzzle
If there was a vial of
Anti-venom that I could
Inject into those venomous
Eyes
And If there was
A clear view of the stability
And if there was a
Definite safety-net to

Catch me as I crumbled
If there was a system of
Dangerous security
A way to keep
Me wanting just enough
To continue the chase
Without losing faith
If I could be given a taste
Only a sip
Of what I ask for
A continuous first moment
Of the scent of you
Maybe then
Oh maybe then I'd learn
To open up my heart
Enough to let my dry
Eyes run.

So It Begins

I've always wanted to be left
By everyone
and anyone who
may usurp my throne.
By any man who wanted
more
than a drowned-out
lyrical melody
to take my place
When I leave him alone.

I've always yearned for
the lurch of a broken ring-finger
The desperate longing
for
him
to want me
like I wanted him
A love-drunk fever

And I wonder if I will
ever
be given the chance to
feel
as crushed
as the snails are
when rain-boots
decide to kick them to the wind

Am I Running

Am I running again?
Racing through terminals,
keeping my eyes on the ground.
I glance at you,
you smile.
But what I really need,
is another dose of denial.
Blame it on the mother,
Blame it on the father,
Blame it on the brother,
or the older sister.
Why couldn't you have…
Why couldn't they have…
Why couldn't he live with the fact that I may just
be a little bit wild.

Flying Continental Pt. 1

I'm flying Continental
And I'm rushing past each terminal
And I'm shackled to these memories
And though I'm swearing to myself I know that
I'm escaping another dungeon I thought I'd cleared

Today is not like yesterday
Nor like tomorrow
Now is now
now is final
Over-exaggerated laughter
Vodka flavored glamour
Let me hide beneath you
Sweetheart promise,
It's only for a little while

Cold lips
Dark tunnel
But it's pulling me harder
Gravity warp in its stagnant portrayal
You've done it this time
And I can't keep from slipping

and I know she said hemisphere
But all I heard was heaven
I've never felt so comfortable flying
But I think
I think and I think
Then I wonder
A near-death experience
Hover
Breathe, you can't let your mother down
And I shiver
Could it have been
Could it have occurred
Is it possible to mentally pull yourself out of the under
But I couldn't breathe
Lungs stuck in despair
And I couldn't move one muscle
But I'm still alive

More than ever

2 Returning to Face a Different Side of the Same City

Reeling on the West Coast

[September 17, 2011]

It's Happened

Don't pretend you're stupid
When you know exactly what you've done
Who would've thought
Angel
would fall in Love

It's happened
I've fallen and the world is looking up
I've found that broken body
That's here to lift me up.

And when I thought I'd lost it
You were there to bring me back.

And when I cried for mercy
Your wisdom shut me up
No, there's nothing more I ask of you.
There's nothing more I'll ever need.
You've given me a chance to see the light,
and I'll hold fast to that.
I'll hold fast to that.

And I can't say

And I can't say
that I got what I wanted
OR at least I didn't want this feeling
I'm forgetting to breathe
And that's just a habit through the hazy moments
But I'm remembering because you say it
And the world has never looked like this before
Time has never allotted such detail
But in your eyes I've found the method
To unlock all that I've ever wanted
Maybe I should be like water
Or test the ground of a lovesick summer
But you meant so much more
Then my silly lyrics would ever be able to unfold
And my thoughts are swirling…

I Don't Have to Be Near

I don't have to be near
to feel all that you've given me
From the moment I picked you up
You've been contemplating why you met me
And if it's meant to be
Baby let it be
Baby let it be
When you doubt what you've seen
Bring it back down a level
Bring it back to me
And baby you can learn
Around you I found no fragments
Nothing difficult
IT was easy
And when I left
There couldn't be more things
Telling me <u>not</u> to leave

You think it's fun
To watch the unbreakable fall to her knees
And now I can laugh again about it too
Because I know you'd give all you had
To be lying under my dreaming tree
Miles away and I can still feel your embrace
Fell into you and now I know there won't be another one for me

Freedom and now I'm free to feel it all
I left my key
And I find that you are
Written in my destiny

Don't worry baby
There's no need
I've gotchu from now until I see you again
And you can feed the fire again
The bumps in the road
Are only artificial
As we come into our own know
That I'll be waiting on the other line
To learn just a moment more

Remember Hudson's Bay Company
As we watched the shoppers smile in awe
Tranquil and complete
The bed we ruffled as
I embedded you in memory
And couldn't have gotten any
As I look back at these pages of love letters
I read aloud to you a dozen times waiting to see you recognize
How bout the two of us
Walking hand in hand
In the darkness under the highway that hustled me into
Town before I could duck or turn away
The day I let you rest in my lap
Or when I played "Somebody's Baby"
And you agreed and told me I could be yours
That night in the pub
You watched as I read the lonely books on the ransacked shelves
IT was then that you truly feel
in love with Kali Rae
There were countless moments
where I for once felt like the painting I've always wanted
to be
Because before you came it
was so difficult to feel alright
being me
And when that Seagull calm
And collected nervously
Was tempted to come perch on
my finger I saw you believe
You don't need to try so hard
Be what you wanna be
I'll be waiting—and it won't be
long until it is you and me
forever babe
Bound up in beauty

I never knew the power
I possessed until I bought a
One-way ticket to leave the
have-tos behind and find me in
watching you finding you
and so it's true
you and me together babe

If only you knew

Notes from Inspiration Point

A painter named Jonathan
Just arrived
We spoke for a moment or two
Told him we were of the same
Crew
I keep trying to leave this spot
Or to say that what my mother told me isn't true
But I can't help but notice
That this day turned from
Gloomy to sparkling blue
One day, I believe very soon

Birds: September 18, 2011

And when it all seems to fall,
I'll wish upon a fallen lash.
I am late to work again,
of course.
But late is always early,
when I'm working at this speed.

And Julie sits in the seat beside me,
and she's beautiful but God won't let the world see.
She hears differently.
She hears it all,
just like me,
But she asks the questions,
while the others just listen.
They just wait to be seen.

Birds have become a theme,
as the past few months unraveled so eloquently.
And I do not wonder,
why they stare intently back at me.
And I do not hesitate
or stutter
because nothing can astound me now that it's all over.

DR. FIASCHETTI (M.D. PSYCHIATRIST): OCTOBER 12, 2011

Dexedrine (See Appendix A.)

Crashing down in November

The coast is magical today. It's October in Southern California, and I'm driving up Pacific Coast Highway from my apartment in Westwood. I have a photo-shoot on the beach in Malibu. The photographer stopped me while I was running with Stella one morning. He was clearly not hitting on me. I could tell by the businesslike approach and the upfront details on payment.

Having been on several shoots where things seem professional and are anything but, I am more than hesitant to take him up on his offer. But after carefully scrutinizing his online presence, I find him to be exquisitely professional.

He is a writer too. I figure I would check him out. We'd chat online about the shoot for weeks. And he is eager to make me feel comfortable. He is also an author who studies Joseph Campbell's, *The Hero's Journey*. After finding out we have this fascination in common, he reveals that he'd like me to be a part of a project; a project structured around *The Hero's Journey*.

He has booked out the entire beach for the shoot. Meaning he has a lot of money to spend on today's shoot. I feel special being asked to model on the empty beach. This particular beach is hugely famous. It was well known in photographers' circles, novices and professionals alike. There are caves at this beach that produce striking natural lighting of any object that come between it and the viewfinder. Any subject transforms into an Ansel Adams masterpiece, due to the beauty of this natural sanctuary. I need the few hundred dollars, and he needs a model. I don't have an agency, nor am I focused on modeling.

In my naiveté of the process, I throw a laundry basket full of outfits in the trunk of the Range, take all of the makeup I own, which isn't much, and pack a few pairs of boots. It is a beautiful day, and it has been a long time planning.

Pepperdine University looks incredible perched atop a lush green hill that drops significantly to reveal the sparkling Pacific to my left.

So that's Pepperdine. I'd love to have gone there.

I never even thought outside of the one school I knew I would attend. It wasn't a question. I'd be like my father and his five siblings and their parents. It ran in my blood.

The hangers of clothing clang against the plastic containers in my trunk. It's annoying, and it's putting me in an odd trance. I stare once more at Pepperdine in all its bright, white glory and then over my other shoulder at the ocean. The hangers rattle once more, making me shift my gaze forward.

Oh shit! Red light!

I stamp on the brakes. Pedal flat to the floor. The car doesn't stop.

I'm sliding, closer and closer with each milisecond, to hitting the black truck in front of me.

No!! I can't afford to fix his truck!

My foot is hard on the brake, but the Dodge Ram stopped at the light is coming closer and closer…

Boom.

I hit.

It's a low thudding sound, metal on metal, smashing into the back of the truck. It's like the drunk boys crushing aluminum beer cans on their heads in high school. The force of the collision throws my car under the lifted truck like a crumpling can. Each moment my car's being crushed a little more under the weight of the truck. My car skids to an almost stop under his, but the momentum begins to move his truck. Now, my car is crumpling in on itself because of the inertia of the crash.

Adrenaline kicks in:

Get out of here, NOW, Kali! Bad situation. Get out!

The driver of the truck is revving the engine to try and break us apart. Each time, I scream as the wheels spin viciously close to me. Several bystanders have come running over.

It must be bad.

They're waving their arms to stop the driver.

I'm screaming inside the car, but no one can hear me within the piece of metal. I'm stuck inside a tin can being put through a trash compactor.

I can't die like this. I won't die like this.

The man in the Dodge is trying to turn his car left, and, in doing so, is unintentionally now dragging my car like a cat toy underneath its steel frame. I can't get out, but this is becoming deadly, fast. The hood of my car buckles.

I'm done for.

Just in time, the cars stop. A muscular man, younger than my parents, opens my door. He grabs my arm and pulls me out. Then he reaches in, shifting my car into neutral. Traffic whizzes past me on the highway, but I'm alive, freed.

He yells over the noise of the traffic, "We've got to let it go! It's too dangerous."

Having made it to the sidewalk, I can breathe a little.

What just happened?

Traffic is not slowing, and this could cause real problems on the Pacific Coast Highway. A couple of auto mechanics from the gas station on the corner have run out into the traffic to try and bring the Dodge, with my Range in tow, to the side of the road.

My car is mauled in the process. It's terrifying to watch these men work alongside the steady stream of speeding cars. The wind from the ocean smacks my hair into my face. Finally, the man looks over at me.

"Oh my God," he says, one hand on his hip, one running through his hair. He wipes the sweat off his brow, breathing heavily under the coastal heat. "My God."

"Thank you," I say meekly.

"I'm so glad you're okay. I've never seen a car crushed like that," he laughs nervously. "Wow, you're lucky."

"Thank you for pulling me out," I say.

He shakes his head, "Look at that. My God, you're lucky."

Turning to face me, he says, "You were saved. That crash wasn't…it wasn't survivable and you're standing here like nothing happened."

He stares back at the two mating vehicles. The entire front half of my car is completely enveloped by his. It looks like a paper jam. The sound of the metal dragged over the asphalt is nearly deafening.

"And my car doesn't even have a scratch?" the man says, almost disgusted, "Thank the Lord. Thank the Lord that everyone is okay."

EMERGENCY ROOM: NOVEMBER 2, 2011

Emergency Room Visit
NOTES: Seen after MVA
FAMILY WAITING: No
OUTCOME: Discharge
LOCATION: Home
CONDITION: Satisfactory
CHIEF COMPLAINT: Neck and Upper Back Pain, Head Injury Without LOC [loss of consciousness] - sip MVA x 1 day ago
DIAGNOSIS: Acute Neck Pain, Acute Back Pain, Tension Headache
PRESCRIPTIONS: Acetaminophen-Codeine
OTHER: soft collar for neck
CUSTOM NOTES: You were seen in the Emergency Department today for a headache, neck pain, and back pain, after having a motor vehicle collision yesterday. At this time there is no need for emergent intervention based on an examination done here. Because of your neck pain and stiffness, you were given a soft collar that you can wear for comfort. Over the next few days the pain and stiffness should continually get better. If you should develop new symptoms such as nausea/vomiting, worsening headaches not controlled with pain medication, or you should have any worsening of your condition or any other concern, please return to an Emergency Room for evaluation.

DR. CALVIN (M.D. PSYCHIATRIST): NOVEMBER 18, 2011

Xanax (See Appendix C.)
Adderall (See Appendix D.)
Depakote (See Appendix B.)

November Notes

[November 24, 2011]

She's Smiling

In a different country,
and the dramatic ending.
She falls.
She's staying,
She's smiling.

You could have given back the key.
The one I conveniently placed in your wallet.
You could have shut me up,
you could have shut me out,
but instead you left me to my own devices.

And I swore to the world around me one night,
in my hometown, overlooking my desolate life,
sparkling like Blue Heights.
You took me to new heights
and I swore to believe in magic,
That I'd stay searching for my way back to the Northern tower,
where I found the moonlight
casting the perfect shadow, of wonderful dances.
And she's laughing.
She's spinning.

I could've warned you,
I didn't have to book that flight
back home.
Where I had nothing more than an empty undertone.
I could've curled up beside you,
watched city lights turn indigo,
and couples skate on glazed-donut streets.
we could've danced all night.
Thrown the suitcases to the floor,
rolled around in the clutter of clutter
strewn across your living room floor.

Lined In Gold

Every page is lined in gold
An attraction only to enclose
The millions of lines invisible
Swore to myself never to disclose
Swore to the sun's partner
Luna's creation
Never let you discover

If there was a vile
Anti-venom, I could've poured
Into those eyes that stole my light
Maybe, just maybe
Your warmth could melt the icicles that inhabit my room
My room...it all happened too soon

And if I'd found the courage
To rip away
Those disgusting fingers
That smothered me into my hideout
Left me imprinted-severed
A tweaker with a graphic design ever
Left me a broken piece of paper
Needing somebody more than ever
Then maybe I'd have some place to begin
But for now I've got messy feathers
And my getaway let's departing
So I must keep up the running

Just one more laugh
One more glance
The stars, I promise
They'll come dancing back
Twinkling gems down my lashes
Shattering the drought with feverous passion
Unshed years, anticipated, but never to come, tears
My false reality will come undone
The flood gates will open and down my face they'll run
Let them fall into your lap
Fall into
They've soaked your sweater

Overrun their self-constricting container.

Linger

I linger between the tangible and the incomprehensible
And I enjoy the feeling of flying day after day
And I even blast music with the wind down
No just in these lyrics on paper in a shiny cliche down Sunset Blvd
But on quiet streets in my hometown
The bubble town of Newport Beach
Los Angeles is a haven for have nots

And so I do not belong
Because I house a million "haves"
Yet I still have yet to find my better half (the one)

That's alright though
I don't search too hard
Usually they fall into my lap
Especially the worst of them portrayed as the best
And don't tell me I don't like to be alone
Or better yet that I can't
Because actually my favorite place to be is inside my nook
With my guitar, my keyboard, my Stella, and a sheet of paper
A pen would be nice, somewhere, found, on the floor, in this uprooted space,
But I could always write the lyrics in my mind
Most of the song resides in me, but I forget the ones that fail to compliment my journey
I don't forget those
As I forget those who betray me
Or those who don't understand the world I walk in

I can tell you this time
Just this time
I want to cry
I don't want to hide behind
And I won't hide the tears that tears that fog up the all-too-flat world of a room
As I drown in the bliss you've uncovered, what you've excavated
The feeling of devastation
Having found myself turned amidst ashes
The harassing bliss of having clutched and watched the diamond of your eye

Lost in the abyss
Finally caught up in someone else's

Flying Continental Pt. 2

I've been flying Continental and my luggage failed to make the cut
I've been stripped down to nothing
But nothing mocks me all too much
As my nothings become the everything you've got

There are a lot of things I would do,
things that I would say,
Admit to You
I'll apologize before the sun goes down tonight, I say
Now I understand it falls like this
out of grasp
every night
I am running too fast.

If I could ever press record
Maybe I could press resume
And If I never slipped on reflections
Or the heat creatures
Morphed from the asphalt into my memory
Etched like a sharpie
In my mind
intertwined
with lyrics, stories, songs, and the benign
Maybe then maybe…

Disregard the color of the chemicals
Swirling down the sink
To forget the pain in my chest
As I dig deeper into a sandbox belief
That the sand would somehow bring relief
A place where I could rest my broken leather, feathers, tear-soaked sweater
on you empty heart, maybe that would be a start.
I could find a place where forever
Lasted for ever and ever

I'm flying Continental
And my luggage didn't make the cut.

EMERGENCY ROOM: DECEMBER 15, 2011

EMERGENCY ROOM VISIT
FAMILY WAITING: Yes
CHIEF COMPLAINT: Flank Pain, kidney stones
DIAGNOSIS: Pyelonephritis
PRESCRIPTIONS: Cipro 500 mg 20 (twenty) tablets 1 tablet by mouth two times a day.
(See Appendices F, E, M.)

Winter 2011: Handing over the Key

Above a square or dreams, lights, and shopping sprees.
Below a horizon of colors
A couple sat.
Neither beyond 20,
One looked up at the horizon and gasped.

All those years before
Looking up had revealed grays or brownish greens,
This time the light from the sun
Distinguished each brilliant shade,
Developing a spectrum
Far beyond gray.

The day the world fell at her feet.
She handed over the key
The world unlocked itself.
You won't understand until we are older
She smirked and her eyes seemed of the unforeseen.
For the silver key unlocked nothing tangible
but rather vaporous
in its vast incomprehensibility.

She got what she wanted
Now, hop back onto the plane and leave.

I never asked to lose myself
But I've forgotten to breathe—
And your presence brings this back to me.

Landed in Los Angeles
Lyrics envelop the mind
devouring stability.
And the endless How of palindrome exercises:
Armana equals Kali squared, when I am left to my own
Without a key
Devices reveal superficiality when writing should be created
by happenstance and recordings never meant to be replayed.

Found a feather,
It's dated 11/11/11,
Same as the recording that found its way

Into her iTunes that day
She listened to her own voice say, over the twinkling of an unlocked car
door, keys in ignition:
ding
       ding
            ding
                ding
"I guess I'll just wait then."

January 8, 2012

Location: Newark Airport

Time to pull it together and realize you do have it all, and it's the thing around your neck.

Can I just close my eyes and wish it well we had the most incredible journey More to come.

I feel like I need to go gnarly in depth about the trip from LA to spend New Year's in Canada and the last couple in New York, but you know what, I think it's unnecessary.

XO Kali Rae

Inspiration Following Trip #2 to the 6 Side

[Winter 2012]

Queen Street Anthem

It just feels right in Toronto. It is like the entire universe is yelling at me to be there, to stay there. And, in this same way, Andriy makes sense. It just works.

Rolling and finding new worlds within Andriy's world, meeting new people in new countries, with new ideas. Everything is fresh, exhilarating, all of the time. Most of all, I feel empowered emotionally. I don't need validation from anybody. And I know that the world is my oyster, that love is all there is and that you sculpt your reality with each and every thought.

L'amour est Chance, Decouvrir la Nouvelle

Michael Jackson's family trust, thrusts my Prius into a lurching,
morning rush.
The circumstance, circumvents the idea that idealists are not realists,
I find the circumstances of this preemptively dated (as if anticipating the
Hero's Journey
unraveling within my, equivalent to Hell, academia approach)
inscription; wedged between the account of discovering that this year, "It
was
going to get louder."
Intersecting. A pattern emerges.
Fucking patterns.

The writings on the wall took form in a rose-patterned leather,
Lavish and Squalor. Raven and Drake; the Canadian shop owners. Toronto's
Andriy
Phillips Square seeped into me, along with Raven and Dale's ramblings.
Their philosophy on artist interrelations and charming insistence on the
comfortable they thought I needed
tickled my throat and dwindled,
The conversation to persuade
Progressed.

I want to move to Canada
I want to move to Canada
where signs do not cease to surmount symbols
Where signs become more than insignias of could-have-beens
Where the vertical beauty of the CN Tower, on the sunset, displays an
unyielding,
Alien light show.

There's more out there.
The Canadian National Tower and that something brushed noses.
Once Upon a time,
It sticks higher than the rest
Or used to, My Canadian and me laugh about the fact that it used to have
the largest
Dick, now only third,
After Dubai and "some Asia twin towers" stole its erection.
Nathan Phillips Square.
Jack Layton's memorial still fresh

Left chalk phrases in all languages on the crisp cement
Unity in a Universal argument.
One Love.
Rather than the usual distinction between one tribe tribe and another.

I lose it sometimes, amuck with inconsistencies, and the Universe strike me in the
Forehead with a couple stones,
They're SIGNS,
SIGNS everywhere.
SIGNS pointing me toward Toronto.
I left my feathers there...

Reve de Couleurs
Clipped from a magazine article in the Maple Leaf decorated aircraft
As I departed.
"Dream" or "to see in color,"
This is written underneath the signature of a fell Taurus.
A crescent moon and star as well as the traces of doves and a halo'd girl.

In remembering that trip,
I remember to eat.
And to Swim Good, a favorite song,
Which holds my heart
As well as the heart decorating the I,
In the title of the song.

Looking through the avancé
Scribblings of self-discovery, taped into a rose-leather life of its own.
Today,
I push
Toward the side of my office space
The Grammy-winner looks to strike a deal,
"Will Wednesday work for yah, Kali?"

Thursday would be better.
The Weekend is from Toronto. He says:
"Not on Monday, Tuesday, Wednesday, Friday, Saturday, Sunday, but on
THURSDAY..."
Until I find my way back to *The Weekend,*
I will schedule the meeting for Wednesday.
Avoir present a l'esprit

Mixtape Messages

Synchronistic. Coincidental.
The Universal Law of Attraction.
Quantum Physics.
Inversions, reflected...
Cathedral of mirrors.

Painful bliss
Found in painful exposure.
Utter confusion
I couldn't bridge the gap.
Yet sewed it
into the label of my clothing.

Absurdities fall into place
The necessary day's flavor
Snowflakes—
Fiercely fought-against by warriors of the storm,
But cherished by housewives—
It's essential for children to know that differences are heavenly.

Each snowflake its own fingerprint.
Not one like the other.
Many more than 32, so many more than 32 flavors.

"Read me yours again..."
"Came bi momenti…"
"In English!"
"It is in your moments of decision that at your destiny is shaped."

Changing the stars.
I think we did it I hope you don't shed them now.

just because it looks Russian doesn't mean it is Russian. Our tattoos'
typography is a typo.

Phases of the moon spill volumes for those subscribed to *Dailytarot.com*.
Tonight, MTV's, moon-man soldier, equipped with a fishing pole
Demonstrates its depleting presence of self-realization: Zen
Oh. how it's waning, especially tonight.
Empty Vase—the name of the store that the Valentine's Day rose petals,

rose from, withered, while days turned to months, and the love, then shared, turned. Accumulation of thoughts churned within a lonely Theta frequent. The petals are crisp by March.

Dream Hotel— Found The Teachings of Buddha in bedside drawer, "The only way to Heaven is Jesus Christ + Not Buddha, Don't be confused. Don't let them get to you"
The inside cover read.

Similar frequencies.
To Kali, From Drake, Beckett, Elliot.
The book is signed.
The cover is ripped
Not so cleanly, from its trunk. The branches hang oddly in anger. A rigid dispute over what
Must have been a perplexing day of putting self in relation to the World, supposed it is not full of entropy.

To the pink pocket planner
Thanks for holding unimportant necessities.
You provided an image of efficiency.

The World has only begun to show itself.
The World has only begun to show itself.
The World has only begun to show itself.
Unlock the flat note in the misunderstandings.
Unlock the flat note in the misunderstandings.
Unlock the flat note in the misunderstandings.

Did I take the right turn at the fork?
I cannot find home anywhere
The snowflakes are competing paradigms.

And I'm losing myself time after time... Cathedral of Mirrors: Winter 2012

Listen, Mama
Listen!
I hear a violin!
That man in the penguin coat is playing it!
Look, mama
Look!
I hear it
I do.
It's there.
He's playing the instrument,
On the water,
But our minds have been perverted with reality.
Or is it?

But Mama,
He's in the water!
How! Mama how?!

A young girl tugs at her mother's waist.
I capture a glimpse of the drama
From afar.
It's safe up here,
Perched above the scenery:
Early morning seals barking, the only footprints
Trail behind the mother and daughter.

It's safe to see into this child's world,
To walk alongside her in the wet sand.

While up here
It's all so far,
So far away from any pain,
Exclusion,
Lots of love.

I see everything she describes.
But, I remove the 3D glasses after.
Hers are permanent

She lives in a different world.
And
In some ways,
I wish I lived there too.

I hear it loud and clear!
Do you hear it yet Mama?
I hear the music playing!
I feel it too!

The youngster mimics the sound of the violin
In a high-pitched cry
There is a definite emotion within her depiction
The notes are lonely.
Destitute.
Lost.

I remain safe up here in my Ivory tower.
Hidden from usual view.
Inspiration Point, serves as my lair to spy
But, it doesn't hide me from those who look skyward.
This little girl looks up.

I look down and grin,
I wish I saw the violin player still.

I wish I felt the notes,
Saw them scrawled
Across the sky so intricately laid-down.
Con-trails of sheet music.

All I see is grey Mama!
All I see is grey. I want to see in color.
I want to feel color like I feel sound.

She glances up,
I look away.

Glazed City Walk: February 2012

Right on University
Up Queen Street
Left past Nathan Phillips
Square…
And the whining builds
Between lover's arms
Wind tearing at their embrace
The number four.
The empty triangle,
An instrument
For the wind to tear,
and split,
sealing fast the ice into
glazed-donut streets.
Only careful from morphing them
Un-skateable.

That Feeling: February 18, 2012

"That feeling the first time I met you"
God I love you and I love the NO SHOES
"Now we're together and I wonder if you feel it too?
"Welcome to OM"
I spoke because I found him attractive. I shut out when he failed to mirror my transgression.
That doesn't really fit here does it—
Multi-colored, mosaic lamp—
the urgency is lingering at the base of my neck.
Next door I hope the strangers act appropriately, is there a rule regarding laundromats and laundry?
I ~~was told~~ read to LOVE everything even use props to prop imaginings into belief, as I reminisce on the Starbucks I booked my flight home at unenthusiastically, I wonder why nostalgia has to sting so harshly, you're so busy carrying
There is an angel looking out from its humble position, from my view, framed by the wonderful exotic purple and patterned throw framed upon the appropriately painted walls they are orange
I enjoy or rather bask in the insecurity of being so utterly out of place
Marc Jacobs sunglasses
I almost wish I could detach yourself from the angel you cling to swept into my messy bun
Behind the counter I could guess what they were talking about but after dishing out 3.50 in quarters via VISA I'd rather stuff my head back into the books
Every day has some meaning, now that it's 2012. Playing with numbers has never been so intriguing.
Connecting the heart and mind could not be more difficult when the mind cannot separate itself distinctly into a left and opposing right hemisphere
I suffer from the condition
The Beverly Hilton
I blasted "I want to Dance With Somebody" as I was stuck one car behind the rest who had been let through the most recent GREEN LIGHT
I was hoping to make it not get stuck next to the ton of tears to my left. I saw it coming but thought I could squeak by

Promises

The sun beats down hard on the business school parking lot: a stagnant heat. The perfect kind of Los Angeles day. It's in these moments that I feel like a ball of clay baking under the New Mexico sun: being turned into terra-cotta, cracking, bursting at the seams to expand.

I'd been so tense inside Haines Hall. It's freezing in there. Making it onto the platform where my car is parked is like opening the gates to heaven. The warmth is invigorating and calming all at once.

The heat returns the warmth to the tiny muscles that I can't quite pinpoint until they release, I've been holding so tight for so long, clenching everything to subconsciously build heat. I exhale. I only now notice that I've also been holding my breath. It reminds me to take a large inhale again and repeat the process.

I just got the news that I will graduate exactly when I want to, at age twenty. This frees me up to finally live out all of the things I've dreamed.

I've got to tell Andriy! I can go to Toronto now!

"Andriy!" I shout.

"Hey, babe, what's up?" Andriy says.

"I'm going to graduate in a month! It's all set! And then I can come to Toronto!" I say into the phone.

"Wow! Serious?! That's awesome, Kali. Congratulations! I'm so proud of you babe," Andriy says.

"Yeah and then I can come see you!" I say. I am a little disheartened that he doesn't mention anything about Toronto. "I'll be fully graduated in one month. I can't believe it. And I've been looking into that Canadian recording school!"

"That's my girl! Wait…one second…" Andriy says.

I ponder the idea that I will be done with school forever in a few months and slip into the front seat of my new charcoal Range Rover. I pick at the parking sticker, waiting.

"Hey! Kali, I need to get back to work. My boss is pissed."

"Alright, well, I guess…call me later," I say.

"Yeah, for sure, love you, babe!" Andriy says.

Click.

All Right: March 4, 2012:

I'm waiting for a day for it to all be alright.
I'm racing from something that felt so right.
And I'm waiting for you
to come with me,
to take the dive,
because I feel so alive,
So alive tonight.

But it's all a fantasy,
I took the dive alone.
And in doing so,
I saw you wouldn't be there break the fall.
And no, it doesn't feel all right now.
It doesn't feel all right.

Fall away,
I tell myself,
But it doesn't come easily.
I ask myself,
over and over,
night after night,
why do I still
expect you to catch me?
I'm tired,
I'm ruined,
And now I'm falling in love with the wrong guy.

EMERGENCY ROOM: APRIL 14, 2012

EMERGENCY ROOM VISIT
CHIEF COMPLAINT: Right flank pain, dysuria, and fevers x 3 days
DIAGNOSIS: Pyelonephritis
PRESCRIPTIONS: Keflex 500 mg 40 (forty) tablets 1 tablet by mouth four times a day
FAMILY WAITING: No
(See Appendices E, M.)

Mind–Chatter Malaise, Attempts to Reconfigure it

Every moment falls into place. The synchronicity is astounding. Things materialize for us. It is as if I have a magic wand and Andriy has the power to use it.

I can barely take a step into Toronto without stopping to process the overwhelming feeling of love, security, and safety in such an insecure place. We don't even have a place to stay: nothing. But it is perfect.

I float through the days laughing next to him, discovering new places and gazing at the vibrant street-art.

At one point, lost, we get stuck in the middle of the university's parade. Within a couple of minutes, we move from angry and tired, sleeping on opposite ends of a public park, to laughing so hard I cry. We are stuck in the middle of one of the largest parades in Canada.

I can make anything that I want, with one downfall, it will all be made up in my head. My life is a projection of the things I truly wanted at that point. But, when things get tough, due to the impending human nature to want to grasp everything instead of live within it, I get scared.

I try to find the reasons behind the mind-gripping ecstasy that I'd been in all that time, the feeling of falling without ever hitting the ground or caring if I did. There is no ground; it is all malleable.

I fall into this person, his life, his reality, and color it with all of the shades I want to see in mine. He falls in love with me, and I fall in awe with the world. Because it isn't about him; it is about the idea of being renewed. It is the feeling of saying what is on my mind without searching for an emotional safe-harbor afterward.

And if I can't have it when I want it, I don't want it at all.

When I realize that I concocted the entire thing, I put myself through the ringer. I am unable to readjust to the new reality. I cut it off with Andriy like someone shuts down a computer. I short-circuited it, pulled the plug.

I am unaware of the repercussions of living this way, completely naive to them. And it still hurts.

Shutting down the relationship makes things crazier. I run as fast as I can to try and find someone, something, or someplace to take me back to where I felt alive: to the nights I'd never forget in the places where having someone as a friend forever meant so much more than having them as a lover.

I am aggressive in forcing the implosion of this dream. I go out of my way to put a wrench in it. It was all so much, too much to take in. The synchronicity, everywhere, and the gut feeling of just knowing that I shouldn't have gotten on the airplane back home.

When I shut it all down, I thought it'd be like usual. But it was far from usual. I scramble to pick the fragments of myself off the floor. At times, I still fall back into that feeling of being shattered by my mind:

It's fake. This is all in your imagination. Only you see it this way. Andriy is NOT here. He has rescued you before, but he isn't here to rescue you now. He isn't ever going to be here again. This is where the page turns. This is the end for you. It ended the day you didn't cry as he told you he loved you and left. Stop trying to feed a fire that burned out long, long ago. It was surely magic, but now it is dust. Time to move forward. Quick and painless. Erase it...

Why are we so quick to cut ties with the people who once brought us such immense joy? If it is all manufactured within ourselves, the least we can do is realize we can recreate it wherever we are, with whomever we want. Or maybe, just understand that we don't have to be so sad. That this is a manufacturing of our minds, and in knowing that, understand that happiness can, therefore, be manufactured again.

This is the mantra that plays out in my head each day after completing my last semester in college. Each and every day it becomes harder to fight the urge to decide that nothing will ever be as good as the way I remembered it. Nothing will ever compare to the days that turned into weeks, scribbling into my journal and buying airplane tickets to Toronto on a whim.

Losing the Key

It is about a month after graduating that I lose the key: his ring. The one I wear on a long ball and chain necklace every day as a reminder of the ecstasy I felt during our adventures in Andriy's American Apparel button-up sweaters that always smelled so good.

On the seventh floor of the Grove parking, I reach down to grasp the only thing I have left of us. It is gone. I know in my gut as I frantically tear apart the inside of the Range Rover that it is over.

I should check the fitting room at Nordstrom. But, I subconsciously blame myself. And, in too much of a hurry to go back and check, I search under every seat of my car, pray, and go home.

I tear my room apart more than once, and all I find are the pictures that Andriy, Victor, Julian and I took with my special occasion disposable camera. I get to sleep at five a.m. sans Andriy's ring. The only thing that meant the world to me is now gone.

Whether I like it or not, it is truly over. My Higher Self made the decision for me when it pried the last thing I had of this relationship out of my sweaty palm. I let go of the rope, but I am clawing at the air on my way down.

The Rose-Patterned Leather Journal:
April Showers Bring May Flowers...Right? Please?

April 21, 2012

I want Andriy's ring.
I have it.
Where is it?
XO Kali Rae

Fumbling Past: April 23, 2012

And I don't think you've got it down.
That I'm fumbling past it now.
I'm slipping quicker,
Into this midnight elixir.
And you're gone.
I know you found it somewhere.
Dundas Square or maybe the pub
where your eyes
finally noticed
the spark they'd given mine.

April 25, 2012

Andriy is coming. This is going to be the greatest birthday ever.
XO Kali Rae

Take Me Back: April 27, 2012:

Take me back.
I'm racing through
worn out letters.
And
Some times
I remember
better than
others.

Quick to Fall Away: April 27, 2012

And I'm quick to fall away.
Because I'm looking away
I'm looking away.

You didn't have to text me when I got home
Explaining all of the things that I happened to do wrong

I left my feathers far beyond Toronto
And now
when I look in the mirror
all I see is you
and you don't even like me either.

I'll Wait as Long as You'll Let Me

And I'll wait for you
as long as you let me,
It's time to take a dive
into the abyss,
without feeling lost,
without this.
And so I'm letting go.

If I could ever press record
Then maybe I could press resume
Rewind, so novel now,
would then be an option too.

Cold Feet, Dropping the Ball, Wanting to Be Free

Driving down Sunset Boulevard, I pass the giant, beautifully adorned sculptured guitars standing up in front of the first office building on the strip. My thoughts race. I feel one thing burning deep in my gut:

I just can't take the time off. I can't take the time off to see Andriy.

I was just beginning the scary/exhilarating journey into the audio world.

I just finished an internship at a leading music-publishing company in Hollywood, and audio engineering school starts in a month.

I am just getting into the flow of independence and making a name for myself. I am finally working toward a huge goal of mine: writing my first hit song.

I graduated winter quarter, so this is the first time I have off from school since, well, ever. It simply isn't the time to flee to Canada.

What about Jamison? I am so excited to start working with him as an artist. And then, there is Azad. He was right when he said, "Andriy isn't here with you. I am. Just think about that."

Little did I know I would hear this same comment a couple of years later regarding Christian living in Vegas. I seem to have a thing for long-distance, open relationships. They are easier to think my way into and easier to navigate my way out of…

I've got to call my dad and tell him.

My mind insists:

Get it done. This isn't the time to run away to Canada to see the boyfriend who doesn't even live in the same country as you. Does that make any sense at all? Cancel the trip.

"Hello?" my dad says.

"Hi, Dad, how are you?" I say.

"I'm good, sweetie, what's up?" he says.

"I'm going to cancel the trip to Canada. It's just—" I start.

He exhales and cuts me short: "If that's what you want to do, just make the decision and move on."

"Can we get your money back?" I ask.

"No, Kali, we can't do that. If you call them right now they might be able to give you credit to use at a different time," my dad replies.

He sounds taxed but kind and ready to help like he would swoop in at any moment and pull me out of danger. Or maybe, less dramatically, ask the very dreaded question that people ask when they know the answer: "Are you okay?"

My stream of consciousness releases.

"It's just that audio school starts in a few months, and I'm working on new music with this new professional musician guy, I haven't been feeling well, and also Andriy lives in Toronto. I don't think it's ever going to work. I don't know how to tell him, but I think he just needs to understand that I am not married, I live in Los Angeles and he lives in Toronto… And—" I ramble.

"Well, how do you think he will take this? You may want to think about that," he says.

"Dad. I just can't go. I just don't feel right going. I feel like it's kicking up dust that's already settled. It's over for us; he just won't admit it. He's too far away," I reply.

I hang up the phone, liberated. Now it's time to unravel myself to Andriy and see what happens.

Or maybe, not just yet. Maybe I'll just give him all the reasons it's not a good time to fly out there and save the difficult stuff until it's more clear-cut in my mind.

I like to have diamond-like precision in finally discussing with the other party what I've mulled over for so long that it's lost traction in my mind.

When the emotion doesn't cling so readily to the thought of what I'm going to say, then I'm ready to give it a whirl.

Now just isn't the time. Turning up the radio, I blast everything out of my mind.

I hope Dad isn't upset that that was his gift to me and I canceled it…

No time to get wrapped up. I'm not the type of person who can just put a toe into the pool I've stuffed deep within my gut. If I'm going to get emotional about it, I am going to get very damn emotional about it. And now is not the time to break down.

The time to go there evaporated within those seven years. It was never the time "to go there."

In retrospect, it was a blessing. If I had had the ability to stand in one spot and digest the weight of some of the situations I got myself into, I'm not sure I'd be here to write this. If I were to fully unravel the knots back then, I might have been too devastated to continue.

April 29, 2012

Andriy, I just want to make it clear that we are both living our own lives and that we can both release ourselves from any guilt about what had gone on while we were separated. I can't live with the shame of forcing myself to…

XO Kali Rae

April 30, 2012

I broke up with Andriy today. It was the correct things to do. I miss Stella, and I miss my best friend. I miss knowing, so I'm going to change direction.
XO Kali Rae

Broken Promises: April 30, 2012

I didn't want your tears,
but you chose this.
All I did was seal the deal.
You gave me what you had,
and I tricked myself to believe
that you were everything.
But it was only me.
I'm lonely too

Jamison's Place in Noho

I rid myself of the feelings of being tied to an anchor that has been thrown off the deck of the ship, inevitably drowning me, but giving me a minute to watch the slow unraveling before I'm yanked to the bottom of the frigid ocean with it.

"I've done it," I shout, walking through the heavy door of Jamison's apartment. It swishes shut behind me and my guitar. "I told Andriy I'm not coming. It feels right. It just feels right. Right? I mean he lives in Toronto."

"Come in here. I have a mix to show you. I tracked some guitars last night," Jamison shouts to me from his room.

It is the corner room of the three-bedroom unit. The apartment has two other bedrooms, a living room, a balcony that extends the length of the unit, and a full kitchen. Jamison's room boasts a window that looks out onto the side of the building, down all nineteen floors to the streets of North Hollywood.

Jamison (a.k.a. guy who worked at the guitar store who I met when I went to sell my keyboard and proceeded to like his Livestrong bracelet and left with him to see his apartment and play music) lives in the up-and-coming "Arts District," a pretty hip spot. At night the view is beautiful: a metropolitan suburb. It is getting from the Westside over the hill that is a hassle. You can always trace the neon ant colony trekking its way up the back side of the Hollywood Hills into the celebrities' estates. In another direction, the same trail continues off into the sunset, never ending, across the ocean of flatland that is The Valley. The Valley is the place "where dreams go to die," a wise man of the music industry once told me. It is a glamorous slogan if I may say so myself. If dreams go there…*am I riiiight?*

In each direction it is vast and sprawling. Despite the seedy nature of North Hollywood, especially the spot where the subway is located, the building seems to host the newest, shiniest members of the music industry: a heavy emphasis on hip hop and electronic dance music.

"You know Andriy, the guy I told you about? How we fit so perfectly when we're together, but—" I say.

"But he lives in Toronto?" Jamison finishes. "That doesn't seem like a relationship to me."

I laugh. I'm a little too ready to accept disapproval of this relationship. It's like a jewel tossed into my bowl each time someone's shallow opinion on long-distance relationships agrees with my decision to cut ties with Andriy.

"Clear your head, let's get to work," Jamison says and grabs his guitar, reaching around it to smack the space bar on his computer. "Yolo, Kali!" The music begins to play.

He sings along like he always does and it's the equivalent of a boy-band member with a sinus infection. He loves, debatably of course, the worst genre in all of music: teen pop punk-rock. I think "Lying is the Most Fun a Girl Can Have Without Taking Her Clothes Off" is his favorite song of all time and Panic at the Disco, his favorite band. He showcases each track from 2005's "A Fever You Can't Sweat Out" whenever he can.

And together with his discarded black and white checkered sweatbands and the hole in his lower lip from a well-worn lip-ring, he is probably the most unattractive type of guy to me, which is just fine because all I want to do is make good music. He is a great guitar-player looking to go solo.

It's ironic that most of my reason for canceling the trip to Toronto was my belief that I needed to finish "Shedding Feathers," which was written for, and about, my time with Andriy in Toronto.

Anything to Feel Alive Again

I spend months searching everywhere inside and out to figure out if it was love, if it was drugs or if the unexplainable thing with Andriy is just a rush from the bravery it took to run headlong into uncharted territory.

I try doing the same drugs. I try falling in love with a stranger. I try jumping off of things. And then I try blocking out altogether what has happened.

I end up back where I started.

After I relax about it, an even greater experience falls into my lap. It falls there through a series of synchronistic events that lead me to yoga class and back to that night in Nathan Phillips Square, the night when there was so much magic in the air that I knew anything could happen, and things were going to be fine.

I remembered that I control my reality and that things are never as they seem. I can pick and choose what I want and what I don't want in life. It is all a choice. I didn't even have to book a flight home if I didn't want to. Having your emotions validated by an outside party makes no difference because an outside person is not the one feeling them.

If you search for something outside of yourself to bring you to the place of bliss, at some point, with the removal of that external factor—an inevitability because all things change—you nurse a void in its place that stretches and lulls into eternity. I can say this because that night in Toronto handed me what I had been fighting for the whole time: validation.

When you search within, you find it's all a movie. You project whatever you want on whatever situation you want. And that's the beauty of it!

It's a game of balance: of not only playing on my strengths but recognizing our innate humanity. We are humans. We make mistakes, and we are totally allowed to. Without mistakes we'd never make connections and therefore leaps forward.

Acceptance and gratitude are is the only things required to live a happy life. When you're scared, breathe. Tune in to the excitement of the fear with your breath. Accept that you are scared and tell yourself, "it's okay," out loud.

When you try to control an outcome, you're focused on the path you want to watch it form from. Therefore, when the train, inevitably, takes a new path, say a quicker more direct route, we forget to get off at our stop, or we miss the train altogether, too focused on the track we are waiting for our train to arrive on. Letting go is key.

The Pharmacy: April 2012

Drunken Facade people characteristically swing their arms.
Monkeys caught up in the glam of Canon Drive,
Beverly Hills.

The Pharmacy;
empty.
Except for the actual pharmaceutical line,
that winds around the beer and beverages aisle.

I liked that dress in the window.
And I like the drunks on the street.
Why am I in here under fluorescent death-lamps?
Why am I always here?
I should be there.

As of now,
I wait in line,
psychoanalyzing the woman making snide remarks.
"Ha, I heard it's the look now" and then lists off the many vices:
Alcohol, decongestants, caffeine, cold medicine, anxiety pills, sugar…"
Why so condescending?
I turn her way and smile.
I thank the store for keeping the lights on.
It made the destination for drugs easier to swallow.

Stella rests her head on my shoulder.
Driving home,
I find it impossible not to light up,
the entire car with the gleam of my cellphone.
Sadly, the simple, "Hi!"
Lifts my spirits.
I wind myself back up the hill,
the tip of the mountain
to Lloydcrest.

I thank the gate that locks me back into my ivory tower.
Before stepping on each cement square,
lily pad

to get to the hidden keyhole.
I can feel the movement behind me,
but I don't know who's there.
Why is my dog acting so funny?

To the moon that shines as if following me wherever I go;
thank god daylight savings time comes in two days.
I can't stand the dark much longer,
and you alone can only light up so much.

Even Though I Begged to Forget

I didn't know the night I met Andriy that things would become bigger than me. I didn't know that he would take me to places that I'd never been before, literally and physically, mentally and emotionally.

I understand that most of this is my doing, making the decision to be vulnerable allows all of the magic to come forth. Allowing myself to love without limits, opens the space to be loved without limits. And when I say "love" I mean in the greater sense of the word.

I allow myself to enjoy the present, fully and completely, to make decisions without weighing others' thoughts about them. To shout at Andriy that I am so in love with him that I don't care if he thinks nothing of me, that I would always remain in love with him. I say things like this before it has even been a month's time since meeting him.

Of course, I found myself backpedaling. The tattoo sprawled across Andriy's right side ribcage in Serbian: "came bei momenti…" translates to, "It is in your moments of decision that your destiny is shaped."

And it is in those moments of decision my destiny was shaped alongside a Canadian stranger who whisks me off to a foreign place and watches me fall head over heels for a feeling. I'll always remember that quote, even though I begged to forget it.

The Universe: May 09, 2012

Do you think anyone will ever understand?
I know that I shape my own place,
but what happens if it's erased?
Get your angel back.
And your ring.
I could throw up a universe.
I could throw myself off of this universe.‡

---

‡ Probably my favorite line of this entire book.

The First Lesson with Daniel

I start guitar lessons with a guy I find playing a beautiful song on the Santa Monica Promenade. I approach him, depressed and out of sorts, hating the job I am working: standing in the store window to model the store's California-style clothing.

What am I doing? I go to a top university!

We get to talking and he tells me about his successful past as a musician in Europe. He offers to give me lessons. In my naiveté, I believe he is telling me the truth when he tells me he is a nice guy who will work with me at a discounted rate. He tells me he can introduce me to some really "big players in the industry."

That night they will be meeting at The Standard Hotel on Sunset Boulevard. They are looking to scout new artists. Daniel gives me strict instructions to come at nine p.m. and to look nice.

It is an interesting conversation out by the pool of the Standard. One guy was a producer, the other a writer. They boasted about Daniel's talents and his whimsical estate in Italy. I didn't listen much to what they were saying about Daniel, but I did listen to the comments about liking my "look." They agreed that I could "totally kill it" in the industry, especially if I were to go to audio school. I didn't drink and left quite early with a fire in my belly. My lessons with Daniel would start the next day.

I write "Shedding Feathers" the night after the Standard, and sing it to Daniel the next morning. I record Daniel playing it and find that it sounds like a real song. He instructs me to take my hands out of my pockets, to act like a star and: "For God's sake, sing like you fucking mean it!"

The first lesson is in the epitome of a mansion in the Hollywood hills. It's the ultimate rich hippie, hipster mansion. It's a beautiful pueblo-style home overlooking the canyon, equipped with a full grand piano and small barking dog. Daniel meets me at the door. He greets me with a kiss on the cheek and a "*ciao, bella*!" before taking my guitar and bag, ushering me in before him.

My boots clank on the marble floors.

Shedding Feathers: May 16, 2012

I left my feathers in Toronto
Where I laid my body down the night before
That was the first time
But not last time
I would shed a piece of me unwillingly

And I
Don't want to look down
Can't find the solid ground
And I,
Am falling faster
And you're tumbling after me
X2

I'm a sundial casting shadows
But December doesn't bring the light I need
I tried to sneak back
Undetected
But the suburbs offered me to real relief

And I
Don't want to look down
Can't find the solid ground
And I,
Am falling faster
And you're tumbling after me

And I
Don't want to look down
Can't find the solid ground
And I,
Am falling faster
And you're tumbling after me

I would book the red-eye flight
Just to feel alive again
Just to be anonymous
I'd swim between the sea of
New York city's flashing lights
Around until I found

What I'd left up North with you
Because it's all crumbling down

I left my father
In the city of angels
Just to search for someone
that I thought I knew
And now I'm finding
Or realizing
That the scar was there
    before I ever met you

A Scumbag in Sheep's Clothing, Holding a Guitar

The thing about Daniel is that he is never satisfied. And I love it. I love being pushed because I know I can do it. By the end of the lesson each time, he says I sound a bit better and usually invites me somewhere: an "industry" party that night across the street or a gathering at the Hotel Cafe.

"Lots of people you should meet, Kali…" Daniel dangles the event in front on me like candy.

I kindly declined, not wanting to mix up the boundaries with him. "Nah, I'm okay, I've gotta study."

"Okay, you do you, but I highly advise you start coming to every event I recommend. If you want to make it, you've got to put in the effort."

Every lesson following that first one would be less and less formal and more and more degrading. In my obsession with following my passion for writing music, I listen to every word he says, eating it up willingly.

On my twenty-first birthday, Daniel had me driving to downtown LA to record in his friend, Rod's apartment after Daniel stopped living in the garage of that apartment. Daniel was homeless, and I was blind. As a result,

I offer him a place to stay for more guitar/singing/performance lessons in which he tells me more things about my insecurities and how I'll never make it without help from him.

The last night I ever saw him, he was at another beautiful house in the hills. It was the home of a fellow musician he'd met years earlier when his career was in its prime. The guy was now on tour and needed someone to stay with the dog.

Each lesson, Daniel bitched about the rate of forty dollars an hour, saying that he'd cut it in half for me. That I ought to not waste his time with my harmonies that were off-key and under-rehearsed. It was becoming a sick pattern of looking for validation from a homeless, has-been musician without a job.

Then one day, David asks me to celebrate. He says he wants congratulate me on how much I've improved.

After a long night of rehearsing "Shedding Feathers" for a gig he promised at the Hotel Cafe, I pass out drunk on the fluffy white bed David said he'd leave to me, pinky-swearing that he'd sleep upstairs. Daniel provided plenty of liquor that evening, including a bottle of whiskey just for me, how sweet.

The place is beautiful. The view from that room looks across the entire valley. I feel like I'm in a CSNY film. I have my new Taylor Guitar that he helped me pick out. I didn't feel comfortable making the decision of purchasing an $800 guitar without the help of a "professional."

Nightmare in the Hills

A migraine wakes me up, but I can't see out of my eyes. My contacts crusted them shut. I blink feverishly trying to see where I am and why I feel like I've been hit by a train.

Terrified, I feel someone next to me.

"Get off of me!"

"What? You're so tense!" David says.

"You weren't mad earlier this morning..." Daniel chuckles.

"What the heck happened earlier this morning?! I was obviously asleep!"

And then the memory surfaces.

He was whispering things to me. I flinched away from him, not able to fully comprehend my state of awakeness. I kept pushing his hand away.

In a daze of cold terror, I felt him on my leg again.

We were writing a song together! Why was he touching me?

"GET OFF OF ME! I'll call the cops!"

I leap out of bed, so dizzy that I fall onto the hardwood floors of the Beverly Hills estate. The sun is shining through the wall of windows looking out onto the valley. The morning and its dewiness blaring. I scramble into my jeans.

I run into the bathroom to vomit.

(See Appendices B, O, K, M, N, O, P, Q.)

Unreachable: May 17, 2012

And I thought I was unreachable.
So far above,
that you'd never reach me.
But I'll come down to you, I guess.
And I'll lie down with you, I guess.
But promise me you'll leave me be
just for tonight
just leave me be.
I can't fight
anyone, anymore,
I won't fight anymore.

Go Ask Alice: May 17, 2012:

So I said Go ask Alice
Go ask her
You always said that
I could do better
And I'm falling

I felt alive you felt it too
Let's tell the world I'll have it
Straight
No need to cover this up

Sometimes I just want to ride
this wave
into the next dimension
I want to hear the deaf
I want to imagine the sounds
I want you with me tonight
You and me
Bring it up to the top
Take me to the ground
Take me to the ground
Hold me down
I want to feel it all

Play me until I skip
See I'll burn brighter
With just the tip
It's scratching

Pick my boot up the floor
I don't need them around
When…

Law of Attraction

I am at Brandon and Jamison's, and we are watching a show about the galaxy. Neil deGrasse Tyson speaks about the significance of black holes and the movement of energy. And now, a successful-looking older man comes onto the screen to tell us that our thoughts have powerful effects on the material world.

"Think about it, guys," I say and look over at the very high group of guys at Brandon's apartment. "All of our material things were at one point in time only constructions of thought within an individual's mind. The things we see every day are thoughts manifested."

I am taking notes in my leather journal, but I'm frustrated, realizing that the key to all of this is action. The key is to use these equations in your life: to prove this theory correct by using it. I throw my pen on the floor. My journal thuds to the ground. "I'll show you guys. I'm going to go manifest a helicopter."

The roof of the building is my favorite place to go since Toronto.

NoHo17 is a twenty-two-story building in the arts district of North Hollywood or NoHo. It's a town known for a recent influx of up-and-coming electronic dance music artists and hip-hop dancers, as well as actors/actresses looking to make it big. There is an interesting juxtaposition in NoHo for this reason.

Down one street, there's an active crime scene, and the street right next, a brand new parking lot with a Range Rover, blinged-out, tinted and chromed, like it's made for Scott Disick.

The entourage of up-and-coming producers and artists, dancers and actors that live in the newly built high-rise provides an atmosphere of electric creativity. We are all super driven.

A trip to get a fresh cup of coffee in the lobby downstairs usually includes running into someone you know or know of and want to know.

There isn't anywhere you can escape in the community of this building. But the roof is barely touched.

I have been up there several times prior, and it makes me come a little bit more alive. I have felt dead inside since the larger than life experiences with Andriy. Nothing ever takes me back to the same place, not even the same drug. I tried MDMA one after Toronto, making the total count four times. But, the defeat of not reaching the godlike space I had before makes me even more depressed and I swear never to do it again.

I also mourn the time in my life that I, just for once, felt alive. Every moment of every day I try to get that feeling back.

The entire valley is visible from the roof. In the valley, at night, you see across the plains of Los Angeles, headlights like thread-like stars in the distance. It's a long line of continuous light until around eight thirty p.m. when the space in between cars leaves the trail disjointed, but still meandering through the hills and down again.

The world around the building is far away when I'm perched so far above. The words that illuminate the sign above the NoHo Arts district with the newest slug-line to the newest motion picture drama always hold a bit of synchronicity for me. Every time I make it to the roof, someone from the universe tells me I am in the right space. And I receive a message either from my writing or the sign in the distance. Even when the movie poster changes into a "Wanted" sign, there is significance. Things just fit for me on that roof at that time in my life. They fit in a new way but put me in a flow state so that I can reminisce the right way.

Manifesting a Helicopter

I sprint to the elevator, pressing the button like a crackhead.
Click…clickclickclickclickclick

I knew the four roommates would soon be too interested not to come chasing after me, but I need to get in my zone. I am a banshee. I don't care. The door opens, I jump inside and do the same thing, repeatedly smashing into the illuminated arrows to get the door closed and then do the same with the number 22 button.

The elevator is all glass, so I get to watch the city get smaller as I ascend. When it arrives on the twenty-second floor, I nearly smash into the doors rushing out of it.

I sprint down the hall and make it to the "Stairs to Roof. No Entry" eggshell, paint-crackling door. I push it, and the faulty lock unhinges. Success!

There are stairwells up both sides of the buildingfrom which the view through Windexed glass is unrivaled at night, but rather unsettling during the day. This particular stairwell is clearly not expecting guests.

Behind the "Do Not Enter" door lies a sarcophagus of the underground, underpaid, and overworked scene. I climb the cement stairs. The walls are lit up by florescent bulbs. I jump two stairs at a time. The smell of urine is putrid. and stains in the cement warrant questions, so do the empty beer cans littering the different flights. After the fifth stairwell turn, I slam into the door reading, "To Roof."

It opens onto the vast night sky. The door bangs loudly against the metal handrail as I step out onto the metal grating. The hot wind of summer in Southern California hits me like I am a kite and in my mind I tumble down down the twenty-two flights of stairs that led me here.

I have to cross a few metal steps, hollow, with space between, enough to break a leg, for no apparent reason, before I arrive on top of the uneven, sandy roof. There are pipes in several spaces that I can see. But it is dark.

The only light comes from the city below and the floodlights situated in the corners of this seemingly enormous rooftop.

There are different levels of the roof itself, most prominently a big square a few feet raised above its textured and tarred base. It is this area that I home in on immediately.

This is what I came up here for, not to mediate or write about the prior day's challenges and messages like usual, but to take action, to show the four men I am with, that thoughts not only harness reality, they develop it.

I run toward the platform. It is time.

I hoist myself up onto the helicopter pad and begin running the circle like meditation, circumambulating, tracing the bullseye pattern.

"I'm asking the universe to bring me a helicopter, I want it now, and I will not wait," I say.

I repeat this several times over and over; thoughts clearly focused on the one thing I want.

I hear the door swing open and smack the guardrail. My four friends would soon see me at work. I can't see them at first. It is too dark, but soon, I make out their lazy shapes.

I watch the slow approach of the four men. I am fired up to make this event happen even more than before. I love challenges, and they don't believe I can do this. I feel it as they laugh with one another about something insignificant. They are ready to watch their fun friend act like a fool.

I run toward the helicopter platform, asking the universe to bless me with a helicopter. The four boys sit on the platform, feet on the level ground below. Two sip drinks in red cups; one smokes a cigarette. Brandon pops up from the stairwell, placing his cup on the platform's edge. Brandon is tall with thick, side-swiped hair.

He comes running towards me. He isn't saying anything significant, just adding to the noise. Brandon joins in, running with me around the bulls-eye of the helicopter-landing pad. Up until that time, he just thought I was making noise for the noise of it.

Maybe a half a loop later, the bright lights of a spotlight flood the rooftop. We are bathed in light.

I turn my face to the sky, toward the helicopter, arms out wide, palms up. "I told you guys! Ask and you shall receive!" I shout into the night sky.

The helicopter circles as I stand drenched in its white light.

"I manifested a helicopter! I manifested a damn helicopter."

By this point, I'm laughing in disbelief. I feel alive again, the first time since Toronto. I finally stop running. My heart is pounding near attack-rate and my lungs hurt from my panting. The light switches off and the helicopter flies onward.

Brandon runs at me full speed, face in full bro-mode. All at once, I'm spinning in his arms, even closer to the sky than I'd been: farther away from the city lights, closer to the stars.

It's a sincere gesture: appreciation for the value he put on what just happened. Brandon knew that this was something that had to be understood as doable and also that this seemingly inane task was somehow anointed in the way it played out. I find my footing again as he sets me down lightly.

Brandon grabs my shoulders like a proud father: "Kali!" he says.

The three boys overtaken with their own marijuana-induced, cyclical, punch-in-the-shoulder-like jokes, stare at me blank-faced. They are speechless. A lack of words quickly turns into repetition; as it often does when marijuana is involved.

The least smart of the three keeps shouting at increasing volumes: "Dude, you manifested a motherfucking helicopter."

This last time his voice swerves up at the end like a pre-teen. His closest buddy is shaking his head slowly from left to right.

"What the fuck, bro," he says.

Nice.

I overturned the frat boy behavior.

I finally take the time to glance to the right side of me…

There are people coming into the light.

We have company.

Azad the "Producer

A majority of the roof is untouched by the light. One part stays a bit lit up by the floodlights of the helicopter pad, but another part stays completely unlit. It's self-sustainingly dark, only providing the small circumference of light under the East stairwell's entrance.

A group of people emerges from the shadows under the east entrance. All four of us notice the group at the same time. There's a synchronized stare over that direction, followed by a tangible worry, wondering if these strangers will threaten our safety or kick us off the roof.

"Brandon!?" a guy from the group shouts.

"Max! Bro, is that you?" Brandon answers.

"Hey, dude what are you doing?" Max says and looks at me, eyes as wide as saucers.

"I manifested a helicopter!" I shout.

"We saw that," another guy answers.

A few minutes into a dull conversation about money and celebrities, I manage to sneak away to find a seat at the far edge of the roof on the edge of the raised helicopter platform.

As I sitting cross-legged on the helicopter pad, one of the guys approaches me. I can smell the authenticity of his leather jacket. The smell of the leather mixed with his cologne is intoxicating, addicting: some kind I've never smelled before.

He is dark, tall and strong, a Middle-Eastern/movie-star-looking-guy. He has on dark denim and those familiar Jack Purcells I know so well and a familiar v-neck white tee.

After a few minutes, he puts his number in my phone as Azad (Producer).

The conversation with Azad is a work conversation on my end. He drops some big names and offers to take me to famous studios.

It is only now that I realize the false implications set about when someone who has never heard your voice offers to bring you in for a session or to join their musical group, or for that matter, any group.

You shouldn't trust anyone who offers you something based on a particular skill (music, in this case) that he has not, himself, witnessed.

It's not about trust, but logic.

If someone is offering you something dependent upon something else, if the skill is not delivered or the agreed upon deal is not made good, the contract should be void.

What ends up happening is, instead, C just wants to sleep with A. So, B was never part of the equation from C's point of view. But it was the entire equation for A.

Asheghetam

A few days later I'm in the elevator with Jamison. I've got my new guitar with me, ready to work. I see Azad across the mezzanine. He is with a girl, a very tall, beautiful, black-haired girl who has the makeup of a movie-star.

Jamison repeatedly presses the "close door" symbol. It's as if he's scared. Or he's pissed-off, I can't tell.

"Jamison!" Azad shouts. His date hurries in heels to catch up to him, clopping on the marble entranceway.

Jamison holds the elevator as Azad enters.

"Kali Rae right?" he asks inquisitively.

"Yeah!" I say.

Why am I so nervous?

I try not to look the girl up and down. She has on gold bangles. Even her eyelashes look designer. A sweater swings around her shoulders, Azad's date looks comfy but nice. I am intrigued by Azad and his manners, and Jamison is aware.

I am too curious about this actor turned music producer with the glitzy date, Mercedes-Benz and million-dollar smile. We start ascending floors; my mind roams.

"Have a great night, Kali Rae," Azad says stepping out onto the seventh floor.

When the elevator dinged for the seventh floor, I'd unintentionally lurched forward behind Azad, almost getting out. Thankfully he didn't see the mistake. It's like he's a magnet. The door closes, and I watch the two walk down the hall.

"God that dude's an asshole. What a dick. He thinks that just because—" Jamison rambles on.

I tune him out by the third negative statement.

Why does the charismatic Azad irk Jamison so badly? And how does he also just hang around gorgeous women and know everyone in the building?

Jamison's negative energy festers in his corner of the elevator.

Bye, Jamison, negativity de-masculinizes you.

It isn't long before I'm going to the same building but visiting a different unit. And it isn't long before my love-hungry "friend" Jamison, leaves a rather upsetting note on my car, warning me never come there again if I'm not planning to visit him. He also texts me not to come to his place to hang out with his friends (he means roommates).

Alert: men, just because you meet a girl first and introduce her to your friends on the same day you meet her, does not give you the power to oust her once she assures you again that you guys will never be an item outside of writing music together.

Jamison doesn't understand this, and I don't care. I only address Jamison's threatening note when Brandon texts me wondering why I haven't come around lately. It is at this point he tells me that Jamison won't be a problem since they kicked him out last month.

Interesting how the bad seed gets sorted out when the time's right.

Indigo Much

I look across the vast roof.

The surface area of the entire roof dwarfs the helicopter pad that is so immense on its own. You can probably land thirty helicopters, end-to-end, on this roof.

There are many obstacles, like air conditioning units, but there is also a vast amount of space.

It's a perfect place to watch the clouds change. The days that the sun shines through the clouds like an opening to the heavens are particularly inspiring.

Many days I go up to the roof to escape the people I came to visit. Other times, I drive to the big building in NoHo just to get to the roof. It is inspiring up here. I know there is more to things, people, and situations when I am up above the city.

I write up there , alone, and tape feathers and trinkets alongside the inscriptions. I have recently liked the task of trying to catch the light streaming across one side of my face in a photo: half of the picture lit up, and the other half, dark, my face always looking distant.

I send a picture of the skyline to Christian and he replies with some sort of text that prompts me to send him back this:

Me: Indigo much?§
Christian: woah, are you serious? I have never met anyone besides my mother that knows what that means. Are you for real?
And that is the beginning of a very complex relationship.

---

§ The term is referring to Indigo Children, but the text was regarding our shared worldview and familiarity of the Indigo Children concept and energy work, that there was something bigger out there: a universal energy field of love and brilliance and that it was our job to tap into it.

June 6, 2012

"Doing it Wrong" By Drake is playing. How ironic. Oh, by the way I ran into someone post picking up my graduation pix and headshots who of course knows Julian, Jamie, Andriy...

But I was so sure
I was so sure I'd fallen
But when I stood up I couldn't catch you babe
What to do
XO Kali Rae

Bill the Retired Film Editor

The first time Bill gives me a tour of his home, I think that it is a calling to work for this man. There are angel wings attached to everything.

I connect with Bill because he recently has been very sick. He used painting to overcome testicular cancer. He was a film editor at Warner Bros. for years but decided he would rather not get dressed every day and instead, built a studio within his Beverly Hills home.

This way, he can edit clips as long as he wants, and as soon as he wants to, he can run upstairs, grab a canvas and paint.

He is an avid painter. And recently, he went on a journey to stay in the homes of the great masters: Renoir, Matisse, and Van Gogh. You can rent out the places these men lived during their most creative years. In Matisse's place, they allowed travelers to make cut-outs and paint on the same walls Matisse painted when he was alive. Now that is what you call a destination bed and breakfast.

Every other picture he paints of me has wings attached to my body and a guitar effortlessly strewn across my naked, except for the blanket, body. But not this one. In this sketch, there are no wings. And I remember him sketching it out because it is when he threatened to take my job if I didn't pose for him.

It is my duty because I am his muse, he says. He even offers to pay me triple what I am making an hour as his assistant editor/audio engineering assistant, just to sit there and play guitar while he plays never-before-heard tapes of The Eagles. Bill woos me with CDs of all my favorite bands, takes me to shoot a music video in my favorite place, Blue Heights, (Bill's friend, the music producer, actually lives in Blue Heights. The lookout is his backyard.)

When I get broke enough, I accept, telling myself it is for art.

It is in this sketch that he captures my true feelings about the arrangement.

The one painting that Bill throws out from the night he finally got me to give in is hanging in my apartment today. I look sad; arms crossed around my legs, my legs bunched up against my body, eyes on the ground.

It's a sketch that he threw out without finishing. So if I squint, I can make my unfinished feet into a magical mermaid tail.

Bill tells me that I am going to be something special and that he is going to help me get there.

When you search for the magic outside of yourself, and you believe someone else can make you who you want to be because they see the light within you, you are asking for trouble.

Bill's Hand

Noooooo. Please stay with me.

I wanna shout to Bill's friend as the last one of the bunch slams the door to their sports car. I hang in the doorway and watch the music producer's car back all the way out of the long and winding driveway of Bill's Beverly Hill's home.

One big-time film producer, one sound engineer, one music producer and Dan (now an assistant to Peter Jackson but previously an assistant, like me, for Bill) gathered in Bill's living room that evening, to chat about the process of shooting Dan's newest film.

Dan had my position when he was fresh out of UCLA film school.

Bill asks me to sit in as Dan dramatically reenacts long days on set in New Zealand and fights among crew members.

The most interesting part to me is that they aren't finished shooting yet, and the trailer for the film has been out for weeks.

I ask Dan about this, against my inner voice's advice telling me to pretend I am part of the fireplace.

Dan explains that the trailer is like a ticking time-bomb: a reminder of the impending doom of the disaster.

"We definitely won't be keeping that date." Dan laughs arrogantly.

For the past two hours I've been sitting quietly on the brick fireplace. I am an outsider in this tight-knit older professional crowd. But I feel weird about it. I am not uncomfortable because I don't know them. I am uncomfortable because Bill seems to have me there as a token. I am paid to be there. This is what sets me apart from the rest of the group. It's weird to be paid to attend a friendly gathering like this.

It doesn't help that Bill keeps looking at me and winking every so often. In my head I see myself retching.

It is a delicate balance of listening to the arrogant man boast, not interjecting, but also not staying quiet for so long as to seem bored.

Nodding in approval is a good idea, I feel. So I do a lot of nodding and smiling, fake laughing till it hurts and frowning when Dan talks about long hours and difficult actors.

As the guests leave, Bill mentions that he needs me to stay a bit later than usual so that we can go over some things for the art festival.

I've been there since ten a.m., and it is close to ten p.m. now. But it will make for a good paycheck. I still have to drive all the way back to Noho. I am not excited about chatting with Bill any more than I have already.

It's exhausting to stay in the space between holding my ground against his constant advances and derogatory remarks, but also not coming off as a cold-hearted bitch when the guy just wants to be a man again. It is taxing.

I lose myself in trying to lose him.

Bill locks the door as the last guy leaves. "I have gifts for you. Come upstairs," he says to me.

His comment brings my attention to the dress I'm wearing that day. It's pink, a tank dress, but its tie-dyed portion flows all the way down to my sandals, which I picked after several minutes of scrutinizing another pair.

I always want to present myself well.

Is it too playful? Have I caused him to feel something he shouldn't?

My body stiffens with dread as I try to figure out why he is acting oddly.

Maybe I should just wear long pants every day.

It's been over ninety degrees the past week, that would be, quite literally, hell.

I wage a blame war on myself as I slowly walk up the stairs lined with framed pictures of Bill and various celebrities.

Bill sits right next to me on the sofa upstairs. He recently asked me to start working mostly in his room upstairs. He does have a desk and computer up there. And a couple of sofas, so it isn't that weird.

And then it gets weird.

Bill begins by talking to me about pleasure. He asks if I have ever been pleasured fully and completely. I take everything as a metaphor so I say that I haven't. He explains that he doesn't have any testicles due to the prostate cancer he suffered a few years back. He explains that he isn't able to do normal things in the bedroom anymore, but that he knows how to pleasure a female.

Once again, I, out of my mind, think this may be some mental metaphor. I think he means that he can see deep inside the minds of women and pleasure them intellectually. I know it's ridiculous, but for some reason, this is how I make things make sense that night.

He scoots closer.

I look down awkwardly.

Do I move? Do I move? Will he get mad?

I scoot over without trying to, but he grabs my thigh.

"You are worth so much, such a special girl. I can show you that," he says.

I am scared stiff. Will Bill fire me if I run? My mom likes this job for me.

I allow his hand to stay there, very uncomfortably, as I try to figure out how to leave.

Is this normal? Am I just overly sensitive?

I don't want to be fired, nor do I want him to think I am not grown up enough to understand what he is saying. His hand moves, gross, gross, gross.

As a mere reaction of disgust, I jump up.

"Okay, I need to go. But, I'd love to talk later." I stumble as I unplug my laptop charger from the wall and haphazardly gather my sweater and water bottle, leaving my cell phone on the sofa. I have to come back up the stairs to retrieve it.

It is bad.

On the way home I wonder if I should quit for his sake.

Is it my fault? I don't want him to feel like he made me feel weird.

It's totally fine, whatever, things happen. I had a dress on. You got excited. Your hand slipped. I get it.

I have to fix this.

On the drive home to the valley, I realize what happened.

The next time I see Bill, he tells me that the reason I am not successful is that I haven't lived enough.

That comment is probably the funniest and most ridiculous comment I had ever heard. And that is the end of whatever odd position it turned out to be. For instance, he signs the emails, love you, or miss you, my angel.

I think he is just a funny old man, but when Ben after we had sent him a proposal for a documentary film and he answers that Ben thinks we are "great together" I know it is time to cut the ties and run, quickly.

He paid so well that it is difficult to leave. After a few too many last-minute emergency requests from him to work, meaning to show up and talk to him, I know I am being used for my sexuality and my partnership, not for my brain. I quit.

(See Appendix R.)

Uncomfortably Numb: Spring Turns into Summer

Uncomfortably Numb: June 2012

And I've got a feeling
that all I need,
is a bottle of Jack
and a worn-out tee.
Or maybe a man
That'll haunt my daydreams.
Because
I'm drifting away
And your fingers have slipped
through the cracks in the sky
I'd hope we'd mend.

June 18, 2012

After watching several public figures succumb to our time's inability to recognize pharmaceuticals as the killers they have become, it is difficult to even think people don't recognize this as a problem. With the continued shootings, all by individuals of the same age range and with the same unstable mindset brought about by misused prescriptions, it really makes one think. How is this not being addressed?

A lot of this stems from people not understanding that this isn't someone else's problem.

XO Kali Rae

Not Just Yet

Not just yet.
Don't close the door
behind you.

Not just yet,
I'll fall this time,
You'll always have me,
not now,
Don't say goodbye.
Not just yet,
I'm not ready for this yet.

How come you let me run?
I've never been the one,
to slow down
to look back
but I'm craning to find you now.

Time Code

It doesn't bug me that you're prying.
But it kills me that I'm seething.
If you knew all I'd done,
I would have no one
to believe me.

And I could love you like no other.
And I could give it all away,
I would dance and laugh and bring you lightening,
but I've given it all away,
left it behind,
for another rush.

Signals are passing.
Time code is flashing.
And you are out there like an island.
waiting for a lonely one
to inhabit you and make you home.
But I'm a wanderlust,
And I've gone this far just fine alone.

I could live forever in hell
Or surrender to what's truly inside me.

June 27, 2012

Location: Coldwater Canyon
So I get to move soon to Noho, and I have a wonderful job and family and caring people around me. And I have Christian, who came to Newport with me today and my boyfriend, Azad, and I'm drinking alone waiting for Christian because he's the only one who knows.**
XO Kali Rae

** Christian approached me during a recording session one day and made me laugh, hard. He quickly noticed Azad's overbearing stance and manipulative ways of dealing with me. And he quickly, without making me feel weird about it, said something. He turned on the light bulb in my brain that a bad situation may be brewing. He reminded me that I was allowed to feel happy and free and respected in every way.

He and his mother opened their home to me. They gave me a place to be worry free: it was an unspoken safe-haven. There were never any expectations with Christian or preconceived notions around us hanging out and writing music together. We just liked to be around each other. Christian made me feel safe: lighter. He allowed me to escape a potentially dangerous situation with Azad. And, to this day, I feel strongly that Christian and his mother saved my life in more ways than one.

My Ties: June 27, 2012

I'm drinking alone.
Waiting for him,
'Cause he's the only one that knows.
I'll keep waiting
And I'll keep running away.

Because
I like my ties weak
And
I like my drinks strong.
And I'm fine,
really.
I actually like,
Drinking alone.
And I'll continue to,
Because I don't have
a "you"
to succumb to.

I'd love to rest my head.
And I'd love to come back to bed.
I'd love to take a breath,
Exhale
Inhale
A faded, smoke-break with you.
But I'm clinging
to a past life
love
That I'm fully indebted to.

I must spend my days,
Looking for meaning
in things like paying my taxes
And walking on solid ground.

I'm holding onto it
And I know it's here to stay.
But I've already lost it,
I can't keep up,
No, I can't keep up.

So, I'm forcing my heart,
although overdue,
to open up to you.
Love;
to a man who's watch,
Says more than he does.

When I Gave Up: June 28, 2012

But as soon as I shut the door,
you come running down the hall.
And when I gave up,
you gave it all away,
So easily.

You left me naked,
Sprawled-out,
Invaded, berated,
on a worn-down mattress,
with a worn-out blanket.

The way you
manipulate me
Doesn't come close
to what he gave me.
I've become the swan
you tried so hard
To suffocate

And
Now,
I'm back
I'm the black swan
and I won't leave
this world
before my time
ends.

July 2, 2012

July is here and I sometimes wish it was a different year or maybe a different hour so that maybe I'd feel a bit different or maybe just a bit less torn between me and the You I'd wish you'd be.

And I'm falling and I haven't eaten in a week, and the hunger doesn't bother me because I'm so afraid of the nightmare I had while having to listen to your late night murder shows and your mother's warning to me as "a nice girl" not to readily "come into a place like this." (See Appendices I, N, H.)

Later that night I notice a framed photograph of the original Twin Towers in Manhattan hanging over six stacked mattresses that Azad said he kept for his sisters who are doctors, explaining the shelves of books on cadavers. They are labeled so discreetly I have to wonder what they are hinting.

But it is a nightmare that I'll never forget, where you chained my thoughts up for the rest of time, and I'm left clanging the chains against a mind that won't think for itself anymore.

And in the days proceeding you reveal your true colors: the you that you only let your people, the ones on the other side of those heated Farsi discussions that you always "have to take" and end with usually a warning to me about staying away from people who look like you.

XO Kali Rae

That Time: July 4, 2012

That time I ran the other direction
When you took my arm and I took off
And you came back
And I was drunk
But you were sober
Like always you were with me
But I was all over.

Id: July 11, 2012

My wallet's been stolen
My cards are gone too
My ID meant nothing
But as I thought I meant everything
To you.
He shoved me into a corner,
and you continued to pull me out.
And I drank the nights away,
Worried I wouldn't stay,
I left my body in shambles
to get you to understand.

You Leave Me

You leave me longing when you go,
but you taught about chains
And your country's Asheghetam.††
And told me you heard my thoughts
that that was your power,
To hear me before I spoke.
To manipulate
My emotions through pretending to know
What I actually thought about.
You said you could dominate my mind,
but you said it in a pretty way
and I was taken by surprise
and leaned in
When I should've leaned away.

†† "I love you" in Farsi. Azad taught me this the day he explained that he could not only read my thoughts but control them as well. And, I believed him.

Titanic: August 25, 2012

And when the music dies,
bury me alongside.
I will not go
down with the ship.

Pull hard on the rails,
but I won't give in.
I'm holding fast
I'm finding us,
this ship ain't sinking.

When will I see the light?
I've been waiting a while now.
And I'd like
to come
back home.
Where is that,
I don't know.

My mamma told me
to take a chance
told me to advance
But I'm sliding down
I'm headed back
I'm losing grip
And it's sinking fast.

3 Finding Kali in the Valley

Give It Up: September 03, 2012

Christian is playing his piano.
And I do recall,
a place where we wept as children,
longing for another summer afternoon.
But summer's over.

And I do recall,
all of you
lying next to the only half
of me
I'd let you see.
Give it up

What do you want from time?
when you know there is no turning back?
What do you want from time?
We are at a fork.
And I must learn to love and let go.

And I've never tried.

Trip #3 to the 6 Side

I will be leaving Los Angeles to journey to the place where I found the magic that night in Nathan Phillips Square and remembered why I was put on this earth after all. I am using the miles from the trip I cancelled last spring when I decided to sabotage my own happiness, but in retrospect it was for the best. It seems to always be that way in the end.

Christina moved to New York last spring and left me the most beautiful art installment. She painted these incredible doors. She was studying art history at the university I graduated from last spring. The morning she left she gave me clues on where to find them, just fragments of street names that I had never heard before. I ventured into Hollywood and after lots of asking, the Universe drove right up to an empty lot where the sun was shining through the windows of the doors she had painted and onto the golden weeds that looked like the Moby song.

It was incredible. Anyway, Christina agreed to meet me in Toronto to experience the magic of the city.

I can't wait.

Christian is going to drive me to the airport. He's the guitar player from school whose mother is an energy worker. He is helping me with my first big assignment in engineering school since he graduates a few weeks from now.

He knows his way around. And it's nice to have a friend at the school with such an awesome mom. I am the only girl in my class and school. But there should be more girls filtering in pretty soon. Until then it feels good to at least feel like this guy has my back. He does have two younger sisters who are so sweet and his mother is incredible.

They even have one of those mini tiger cats who sits on the piano when Christian plays for his littlest sister, who is only in first grade but really does have a voice.

Christian and I met in the studio on one of my first days at the new audio engineering school. I stayed after a microphone workshop where we were micing both a stand-up base and a drum set. I was clueless and he had to help me out when I choked not knowing how to test the mic setup on the kick drum. I shocked him when he reached over to scratch the mesh part of the 57 microphone.

He told me later that was when he knew he had to meet me.

The Rose-Textured Leather Journal: Entries from Trip #3 to the 6

September 14, 2012

Location: 50 King St. TN, ON:

"Sail away from the safe harbor. Catch the trade winds in your sails. Explore. Dream. Discover." -Mark Twain

I am rolling tonight and knowing the incredible ability I do have and yet to unleash is a wonder. I will stay connected to Christina weekly. We are all here for one reason and the divinity only grows.

I'm in love w/ this journey, rather pilgrimage, and although I am in the forest, I am only in the forest due to my own decisions that I can't control life= a journey to find the grail.

Music keeps me alive. It is my soul's journey in an auditory incredibility. I find peace when I'm alone and I know why I'm here. Connecting the pieces now will only bring tears.

So lay down your weapons tonight. Simply take a bow for all to come without your fear and doubt. What you see is what you manifest.

Bring the angels down tonight. I'd like to open my mind, to face the abyss.

Never alone, never wrong, unless I believe so. Belief systems are mine to find, the grail to make soul sounds. Awaken me, Mother Mary. I am ready to jump.

September 15, 2012:

Location: 50 King St. TN, ON:

Long night last night. Beautiful in its incongruity. Although I feel as though it solidifies my forest state. I need to appreciate the now. It's so hard for me to fall into the later. I want to love, truly love all that I am. I will. Going out to take a breath.

I want to remember a couple things from last night...

- Union Station
- the birds
- we went to Sushi
- spoke w/Christian because Andriy was scaring me

I still struggle to find time to be present. Christina still is not home. I would really like her to be. And although I have moments of utter confusion in bliss I can't help but want to go back to last year where Andriy was all I had and I saw clearer. I am going to make that change today. Because w/o it I will never have quiet to relieve myself of the trials we face in living after the Fall. To love is to be I cannot write what I do not believe. What I do hold close is the fact that I do not have control which causes a burst at the seams. Who do I want to be other that w/in the melody of a DMB song. Who am I to know that I must stand on this balcony, 17 floors up #1712 and not fly into the beauty of all I see ahead. Why do we cry Van Morrison's "Twilight Zone" echoing profusely I want to wander. What will I find? A broken heart is blind. But I've got dreams to kill and memories to forget and I'm in love with the pure plausibility of changing it all. Change the game changing it all, I'm in with the choices I must make every day because; "It is in your moments of decision that your destiny is shaped."

Tonight I will drink so as not to see the morning come. And today I will savor every last drop of this daydream.

[blank]

A broken heart is blind

September 16, 2012

Location: 50 Stephanie St. TN, ON

Feel like I ruined yesterday with Andriy's dad and sister and family friend because I had to file a missing person's report for Christina who never came home.#

I am in awe of the work that I must do in order to make it out of the forest and into the sun. But I've got dreams to kill and memories to forget.

I'm in love with the pure plausibility of changing it all, changing the game and changing it all.

I'm in love with the choices I must make every day because as Andriy's tattoo reads. "It is in the moments of decision that your destiny is shaped."

Tonight I will drink so as not to see the morning come. And today I will savor every last drop of this daydream. (See Appendices B, K, O.)

I know I could have stayed w/Andriy and we would have had an incredibly explosive relationship. I don't know why I chose to fall into this odd separated state, but I know it's alright. Because everything is always alright. I can't wait for my life to continue to incredible heights.

XO Kali Rae

I haven't seen Christina since this happened.

Search History

One evening, when I was out with Andriy and his family at a Canadian festival, Christina left without a word: all of her belongings and dirty clothes on the floor in Andriy's apartment. After an entire night, day and into the evening of the second night with no response from her, Andriy, his roommate and I were all stumped.

After consulting with my parents about the matter, I regretfully, and in a panic by this time, had to contact her parents to ask what to do at this point. I met Christina's parents a year before at Christina's graduation. They were very WASPy. The owned a country club on the Westside of Los Angeles. And to me, they immediately felt like family. They were familiar.

Christian, however, as an art major, did not get along with them. They did not agree with her life choices, and she HATED them for stifling her. I thought trivialities like this would fall away when someone's life was, assumed, hanging in the balance. But, I was wrong. They were irritated, both angry and worried.

They decided almost immediately to get the police involved.

We all were worried about the same few factors; Christina was an American citizen in a foreign country, she had never traveled to Toronto before, and Andriy thought it was extremely dangerous for a girl to be walking around alone in Toronto at night with seemingly no belongings. It looked like she was kidnapped.

Within minutes of the Canadian police officers arriving, I got word through the police officers speaking on the phone to her, that she was alive. Her words to me were something like, "YOU TOLD MY PARENTS!! WHY WOULD YOU DO THAT?!"

It was only through the search history of Andriy's roommate's computer that the police eventually tracked Christina down. There were internet searches for tickets to Niagara Falls. It turns out, Christina bought a one-way ticket. She explained in rage that she had left her [dirty] clothing and suitcase and backpack to me as presents.

Christina was livid. I was happy she was okay, and the police officers were irritated. One officer kept repeating, to a raging Christina. "Call your parents, immediately."

To this day, Christina won't speak to me.

September 17, 2012

Location: YYZ TN, ON Airport
Flying home today, wish I wasn't
Regretting, forgetting
XO Kali Rae

Just to Feel Alive Tonight: September 24, 2012

I'm shedding feathers
And I'm writing letters
That I'll never have the time to send
But the terminal gate's closing one after the other
I would book the red eye flight
Just to feel alive tonight
Just to feel alive tonight

October 8, 2012

Location: 515 Newline Avenue, Bill's place
Today I take a trip to the canyon. Bill says his famous music producer friend will be there. We are planning to get shots inside of Graham Nash/Joni Mitchell's old place and take shots above Laurel Canyon for my first music video. It turns out that Bill's friend lives on top of Blue Heights, the place Andriy and I watched the sunrise. It is literally his backyard.
XO Kali Rae

November 9, 2012

When I think of what you've stolen,
I embrace that fact that you needed it so bad.
I won't be there to watch you fall.
So take what you want,
and let me walk away.

I can't fathom how lonely you must be
You lost yourself.
And thought it would make sense
to blame it all on me.

You criminal, unchain me
The chains clang.

I Own the Label

The Distressor I'm carrying is super heavy. I look down at the piece of recording equipment that I rented from the audio rental store across from my school. It's a favorite among professional audio engineers.

I heard it works wonders on mixes. The Empirical Labs Distressor will take my group's mix from sounding great to sounding like we all need to be hired by Warner Bros immediately.

I'm excited to present it to my peers and cement myself into the crew as a serious colleague.

I run into a man with long, shaggy, blonde/gray hair parted in the center and a stubbly beard. He has on loose khakis, pin-rolled at the bottom, rainbow sands, an old logo t-shirt. He has his arm around a young boy, dressed like a little rich kid who is staring into his Game Boy.

"Cool shirt!" I say to the kid, staring at his awesome wolf t-shirt.

"Hey!" says the man. "Where are you taking that thing?"

"Next door," I say.

"And why?" he asks.

"We are in competition with the other half of our class for the best mix, and I think this will win it for us," I say.

"You're an audio engineer?" he asks.

"Yes, well, learning," I say.

"Come with me real quick," the man says.

I look hesitant and stop walking as he waves me to walk toward this staircase. I've seen it plenty of times, walking to my recording school, but never had the urge to explore it. It was between the smoke shop where I bought Gatorade and a violin store next to Terror Tours of Hollywood. I am not attracted to the area, to put it politely.

"Okay, look. I own the label," he says

I'm not buying his bullshit.

He continues, but first excuses his son. The gate buzzes open, and the kid pushes through it and runs up the stairs behind the slamming metal fence. "My name is Mark Voss. I own a hip-hop label. Have you met anyone in here yet?"

"No, why would I?" I say.

"You go to school next door! How come you haven't come to visit?" Mark says.

"I don—" I start.

"Here, I'm looking for someone to work for us part-time. Come upstairs. I have a shirt for you. I'll explain what I'm looking for," Mark says.

I am an hour early for class anyway.

The gate buzzes. "Here, gimme that... I'll be careful. I promise," he says and laughs as I hand him the heavy piece of gear. He starts walking up the stairs. "Come on! What's your name, audio genius?"

I hustle through the gate behind him.

What could happen?

"Kali Rae," I say.

His voice is nice, calming, "You're funny, very nervous. I understand, though. You're a beautiful young girl, and this is a crazy city, believe me, I know. My wife is in the movie business. It's hard for you guys."

"Yeah, I've been here a while for school so…" I say.

"Before this? Where?" Mark asks.

"UCLA," I say.

"Berkeley here. That's where my brother and I started the label. But it's been a long time since then…" Mark says.

I feel like it always starts out for me this way. They offer me a job and explain that they are safe, not like the rest of them, either by action or by manipulating situations to sweep in as boss and rescue my damsel-in-distress self.

On a weeknight before the job offer, Mark asks if he can come over to discuss some new designs with me. They have a super classic logo that is widely recognized and sought after. Knowing my background in fashion, Mark thinks I can help him brainstorm a bit to re-energize the branding.

When he arrives, he has a canvas bag of samples.

Perfect! So fun!

…or so I thought. As he unpacks it in my kitchen, he pulls out a bottle of wine, a jar of coconut oil and a bag of almonds.

"You like nuts, right?" Mark asks.

What. The. Fuck.

Tonight's Calichristmas

Tonight's CaliChristmas and this morning I've been sent to pick up what I think the guy said is The Weeknd's guitar.

I am confused by the fact that I thought he was just a vocalist, but I went ahead and picked up the equipment. It was, after all, a treat to get to go to the Gibson warehouse at all.

I arrive at the venue after racing through Hollywood to get to the Gibson Amphitheater on time. I have to battle with security because we aren't given the correct clearances even to get inside the venue. My contact isn't answering his phone, so I call Mark. He apologizes profusely and says he'll figure it out.

A few minutes later he calls back: "Hand the guy your phone, let me talk to him." Mark sounds angry.

After a ten-minute conversation and a couple of cars being diverted from behind my embarrassing vehicle after their drivers whip out their easily visible clearances, the arm lifts and we finally get inside the venue to park.

"Okay!" I say in relief.

I turn to my engineering teacher's assistant, Dylan. He'd been donated, in a sense, for the night and was supposedly a great engineer. I wasn't about to work sound at Calichristmas after only a few months in school without someone there to give me a few pointers.

"You ready?" he asks. And then assures me I am, "You've got this, seriously; it's less intense than they tell you in school. It's the same process every time, no matter the board, no matter the venue."

An hour and a half later, we are still waiting for Mark's friend. He finally pulls up in a rickety, rape-van. He steps out already on the phone, talking with a lazy accent, incessantly. His demeanor is more than crack-like, as he waves us over and then proceeds. Dylan and I are both uneasy now.

"Is this a joke?" I say under my breath.

"Well it is hip hop," Dylan responds.

The night is a debacle.

I end up working outside the venue, trying to record on a console that is installed inside a car. We are instructed to flag down the artists after they perform to sit in this car and record. But, there is no plan in place for this to happen. And the guys who installed the console in the car forgot to install a component that is key to the recording process.

To top it all off, it is raining. I nearly get hypothermia and spend most of the sound check inside the Gibson Theater.

I did get to meet The Weeknd. He is my absolute favorite artist, one of the reasons that Toronto was so intriguing. Right before he steps onto the stage, (I mean, lights down and everything) he is pacing next to me in the wing. He looks right at me, and I can't help myself. It is just him and me. I thank him for inspiring me and am impressed by my ability to come off so calm. Maintaining composure is probably one of my greatest random strengths. I can make it seem like I don't know who you are even if I've been obsessing over you for a year.

It all clicks, looking back at that moment. Mark heard me gush about The Weeknd, that is why he had sent me on the job. It was a secret "shut up about things" prize. I even consulted one of the senior audio engineers at the school I am attending to help me. He was less than excited about being a part and sent his assistant to help out instead.

Mark didn't need me to work. He just wanted to apologize, and veiled it with this event.

Not the One: December 20, 2012 (Christian)

I'm not the one you waited for,
I'm not the girl you want.
I lay out all my weapons down.
I'll leave it up to you.

I told you I was danger,
Why'd you feed the fire?
Now I'm racing through thought-patterned images,
distressed over the unlikely,
absentmindedly manifesting when it'll all unfold.

Christmas Without You: December 23, 2012 (Mikah)

It seems that everywhere I turn I'm seeing you.
No decorations or invitations change my color,
Blue.
And I've been talking about our time like it's anew,
but you're not here,
and I'm still not clear,
as to why I think about you all the damn time.
Why you show up,
Every day,
on my mind.

Why is it Christmas time,
and the only one I want beside me,
Isn't mine.

If I could ask for just one thing,
It's forgiveness from you
and a chance to fall back into your chest.
Because I can't seem to fall
in any other place.

Take every ornament,
I would still be so oblivious to,
the naked tree in my desolate living room.
because
without you,
I can't see the green,
Only blue.

Go Home

You know we can do this again,
for now.
But someday I'll wake up
and I won't need your wine
or your movies
or your 3am calls,
that I never do pick up,
unless I need a refill.

You almost had me.
You almost had me,
but the wine is running out.
And you stuttered,
and then I pictured her.
How she'd wrap her arms around you.
She'd whisper that she loved you,
and she'd want you with her in the morning.

It's time to go now.
You have a empty home that you're neglecting,
and I don't want you here.
I didn't invite you here.
You said we would be working
I don't want you around me anymore.

Go home.
Leave me alone.
I thought you were a friend.
So now it is time for you to go.
Go home.

I told you to stay away
Yet you came rolling back around,
Leave me alone,
Please just go home.

I took you in
and I threw you out.

And you laughed in the doorway
Tried to make me feel dumb.
But I laughed at you
Amazed at what you'd done.
I laughed at you realizing just how small
in my eyes
you had become.
And I really thought you were a decent one.
But you're not my friend.
You can laugh all you want,
all the way home
to your empty palace.

Slinking onto my couch,
you left me no other option
get the fuck out
this isn't a choice.

Love Drunk/I Feel Everything Now

You

You said you were love drunk.
But I kept myself sober.
You said you'd stay like this,
that you'd love me forever.
And now it's over.
And I've been racing back to where it all began.
Losing my reflection in fractal patterns of fucked up.
I wish I'd been there.
I was numb when you said forever.
But I feel everything now.
And this wave isn't passing,
Just keeps washing me asunder,
hemorrhaging into the somewhat pulled together places of my life.
I feel it now.
I feel him too much now.

Him

And maybe it's only because you left me hanging.
Or because he knew I didn't want him all that much.
he knew I was too nice to desert him,
that if he forced his way
in and faked her out,
that she wouldn't tell anybody.
That she'd be a grown woman about it.
But I can feel everything now.
But I can feel everything now.
And it hurts so bad.
I can't seem to put myself back together.
(See Appendix H.)

But I Watched Him the Whole Night

I watch my scuffed-up, faux leather, Steve Madden boots and listen to my heels clanking on the pavement. It is January 1, 2013. Christian and I were at my old stomping grounds: Noho 22 for a New Year's party at Brandon's new apartment.

"I didn't get any sleep last night," Christian says.

"What even happened??" I ask.

"That guy Nico must have drugged you. It was so hard to watch. He had his hand down your shirt the entire night. I slept across from you guys to make sure nothing happened," Christian says.

"What the heck, Christian? Why didn't you push him off me? What happened after that drink Clay made me? I remember going downstairs to that older woman's party—" I say.

"Yeah…you threw up, a lot," he laughs.

"I remember telling you I wanted to go home, that I didn't feel well," I say.

"But Clay talked you into coming out with him, so we went," he says.

"Okay…Why didn't you stop Nico?" I ask.

"He was nuts I think," he says.

"Christian, he's like a little girl. He's my size! Come on," I say.

"It's not like anything happened. I watched you all night, and then you puked all over their carpet. And it was red from the wine. Just amazing, Kali, amazing." He laughs again.

The familiar ache begins to resound deep in my stomach. I feel my real-self shrinking into a tiny piece of anti-matter and self-imploding.

How could this have happened? Christian was with me the whole time!

As if reading my thoughts, Christian says, "I'm pretty sure they drugged you, because you were totally fine. And then Clay brought over that one drink—"

"Oh! I remember that!" I shout.

Finally!

A glimpse of the night shoots across my mind and dissipates, "But not anything else," I realize.

"Yeah. All I can say is those guys are not your friends, at all Kali," he turns to look me right in the eyes.

"Thanks," I say.

We've reached the outer security gate to my apartment. We'd only been a block from my apartment.

"Why didn't you just take me home?" I ask.

"Yeah, okay, Kali. So it's my fault. Dude, I was up all night," Christian says.

Christian pushes past me down the hall toward my apartment. I don't have the energy to be angry. I am too ashamed. Feeling, once again, like I have been stripped of all color and thrown into a vat of darkness. Before I can begin thinking about what transpired during the hours that my mind was off the clock, a splitting migraine washes up my neck. It surrounds my skull and hijacks my vision.

"I think I'm going to pass out," I say.

Christian is already waiting in front of my locked door.

"I'm gonna pass out, Christian."

"Kali!" Christian shouts.

I black out.

January 03, 2013

Bring me to the point where I can shine without a shadow covering the unruly side of my face.
XO Kali Rae

March 22, 2013

I wish the red wine would run through my veins and show me which way
Moses parted the seas. Or at least a place I could pretend was the divine
way to go.
XO Kali Rae

Poems from the Loneliest Summer: Spring 2013

The Loneliest Summer: March 22, 2013

You're afraid to live he said
And he glanced over at me
Take another sip is what I thought
But his light bled over and onto me

I told you I shouldn't
You said you wanted to listen
You said I didn't have to worry
But I fell head over heels
Down the ravine before me
And there's no parachute

And I wish you needed to stay
Or at least that I could feel
Because breaking you
Is not what I meant to do
You let me drink all your wine

If you had told me to get out I would have left
But I'm crying and the tears are spilling into a life I forgot to live.
I'm a little worried that I'll never
Find what it is that I need
in order to survive here
in the loneliest summer.

I Was Trying

I was trying to find something in you
I was looking for someone to run home to
After I've been wrong
We could fight and I could kick
I'm only 21 but I've been through you
And I'm ready to prove it
I'm sorry but I'm looking
It's vulnerability that shines really though
I'm numb
That' why I cry
I cry because I'm numb
But it's better than being able to feel for now
Until I can find the light again
And purify my life again.
I was trying to find something in you.

I Swear: March 28, 2013

It wasn't a game I swear it
I apologize
I took you right in
And I spit you back out
Don't expect my call
Don't want to be rude
But I thought I'd let you know
I'm not the one
You can't dress me up
I used to burn bright, I used to be nice

I lured you right in
And I pushed you back out
In the same breathe
Catching your eye was a game
But watching you fall was not the way I wanted it to end

You poured me a glass
And I drank the whole bottle
You bought me perfume
And I lost it in the move
And you gave me a card
That I melted into
But only for a moment or two

Poured you a glass of the wine
That you'd brought over
Then I drank the whole bottle
Before you turned around
In order to be ready
In order to be ready to defend myself from you.

The way I know it hurts hangs over my desk
there's a day circled
its the date I refused to see you.

Find a Home: April 03, 2013

I need to find a home
Whether that's with you
I don't know
I've got a sore throat from singing
And a year of stories without happy endings
And I've been told over and over to enjoy the present
But I'm learning that it seeps through too quickly.

Tell Me Stories: April 09: 2013

To me it felt forever
For you it was just a test
You know that I didn't want you to stay
But you wrapped me in wine
Told me stories, told me lies
And you never looked back
Not once did you ever look back
To see if I was still breathing.

Life Rolls On: April 9, 2013

No inspiration to give
When you're stuck in the same place
When all you wanted was to escape it
And then life rolls on
Neglecting the importance of 'hello'.

I'd Be Lying: April 11: 2013

And I'd be lying if I said
That I thought things would change
And I'm waiting and I'm waiting
And I'm waiting for you to give me something
Give me something to work with
And I'll give you something to claim

When you take and take and take
I don't feel a thing
It's easy for me to see that I'm all for you
And you are all for one
Can we circle around
Bring it back around to one
Bring it back to love.

And it's only 9 o'clock
But it feels like an hour past 3
And I'm waiting for a difference
I'm waiting for a change
I'm waiting for there to be a time where we are just you and me.

So that's where our story ends
But another will begin
Hold you head up
Soon you'll find something new
That will fulfill the promises I've broken with you.

Lying to Myself: April 20, 2013

When I thought
I forgot
And the colors turn grey without looking back
I'm stuck in a moment without life
And I'm drifting past all of the things I thought
were holding me down.

I wish I could cry
But I've gone numb from it all
Take me back to the life I didn't plan
This one seems to need one so bad.

But I know it was alright
To keep on floating in and out of life
And when the drugs stifled my breathe
I'd take a sip and lose It all to the wind
And I was alright
Because fallings always feels so right
And with you on my mind
I can reshape the landscape
That is ultimately
pushing me away.
So I think I'll stay
Basking here in a summer dream.§§

Lying to myself
Lying about just about everything
Looking back until you pull me back to life
Like you did
In that tunnel
That night when I couldn't find my breath.

---

§§ Referring to the event I describe in "Reaching Out, The Hallway"

MAY

JUNE

JULY

(See Appendix H.)

Don't Walk with Me: July 2013

I'm running,
I'm racing,
I'm losing the battle.
I am not the girl you knew,
I wanted him,
And he never came,
You know my heart wasn't meant for you
And it wasn't meant for love.
I warned you,
I told you I wasn't cut out for this.

Numb.
And it's not a gift.
Can you forgive me?
Could it have been
That I fell
in love
with the one
that would be
easiest to break away from?

Can you be my man?
Just until the wine is done?
Just until I fall asleep,
just for tonight, again.

I'm afraid to open the window,
The list may seep out…
But if you open up that bottle
By daylight
I'll be kicking you back out
The door you worked so hard to barge into.
Stay away.
Do you want that?
Tell me if you want that.
I didn't mean it.
I've been grieving
and you seem to see it.

He hurt me.

I left you.

I abandoned the dream.
The nights of ecstasy
and the lights!
The lights…
I left you.
I left you.
And I've been running circles around electric fences,
Blindfolding anyone who tried to find me,
There's a pattern here
of broken locks
and pills
and places.
You said we'd go
before I stopped
untied our laces.

I wake up in a cold sweat, seething,
I try to remember.
The darkness isn't so bad
until my mind starts to wander.
It's the void that eventually tears at me
'Till I'm tearing asunder.
The wave of knowing
I pushed you away
Until you pulled me under.

One day I hope,
I really pray,
to wake up believing,
in more than the sound
of his bitter words
in my mind,
repeating.
And you'll grab you hand
and you'll spin me around
And will run for the fences.
And I'll watch the bruises fade,
And decide that I may
Be allowed to feel again.

Don't walk with me.

Don't walk with me.
I'm not your owner.
Don't run with me,
Don't run with me,
I'll run you over.
Don't lie with me,
Don't lie with me,
I'm far from sober.
And don't try to find,
the reasons behind,
my bad behavior.

You sealed your own fate.
I told you
to run.
But you demanded to stay.

I told you from the start,
I'm not the one you want
to get involved with.
The doors open.
but I'm not home
and you can't save me.
Forget it.
(See Appendix H.)

A Kind Face

I get into Emerson's beat-up BMW. It's so old that the window has a crank to roll it down. My thoughts are fixed on one thing the entire drive to the concert: alcohol.

Emerson opens up about leaving the label Vic built, explaining to me that he was working as an attorney for them. I had always been too nervous to ask anyone at the label questions. I had no idea he is an attorney like my dad.

Emerson texted me only about three hours ago to tell me he has a ticket available to see my favorite artist from my favorite city: Toronto. Emerson remembered how much I loved this particular musician/singer and reached out to see if, by chance, I would buy the sixty-dollar ticket.

We pass by Om Cafe, next to the Laundromats I went to with Andriy. And then, farther down, past the beat-up houses and apartments that line Fountain Avenue.

I wonder if we'll have to buy alcohol at the venue.

I think about the logistics of how he will probably pay for a drink or two, and then I will be on my own. I wonder if there will only be beer, or if there is a way to get an actual drink into the picture.

After forty-five minutes in traffic, on the same route I used to get to the observatory, we park the car in a sardine-like packed lot.

I am ready to jump out and spend a fortune on a cheap cup of beer when Emerson pulls out a shopping bag from behind the driver's seat. Inside are two small plastic bottles of orange juice, one small bottle of vodka, and one small bottle of Captain Morgan's.

"Oh my gosh! What? You're prepared!" I shout. He's surprised by my comment.

"No problem." Emerson laughs, "I wasn't about to be paying for ten-dollar beers all night. We should probably drink here, though, before we go into the venue."

I am already crackling off the plastic seal of the vodka bottle to take a swig. Before it even hits my stomach, I feel the surge of adrenaline. My heart races fiercely. My chest warms up.

Before I feel the burn in my empty stomach, I take another swig, just to test myself.

Emerson laughs. "Wow. I'm quite impressed."

A few moments later, after admitting he has had a crush on me the entire time he was with his girlfriend, typical guy admission, thinking I'm listening, he glances over at me and sees the bottle of vodka.

My mind is in a completely different place since the vodka appeared in my lap. I am elated. In the haze of the thrill, I am overcome by impulses and the low-lit setting of the parking lot outside the Greek Theater. I dare myself, subconsciously, to finish the entire bottle, from the moment I lay eyes on it.

It has probably only been about seven minutes since we arrived, but I finish the bottle of vodka and am only halfway through the orange juice that Emerson bought to cut it. I am in a state of rejoicing that we have alcohol, unthinking, like if you gave a starving person the keys to a grocery store.

"Holy shit. You finished that? That was for the entire night," Emerson says.

"Oops," I say, gritting my teeth like an emoji, hoping to be spared any anger.

"Okay, geez, woman. I didn't know it was going to be like that! Let's go!" Emerson says.

I run off the cement of the parking lot onto a dirt path leading up to a deserted restroom.

Emerson is calling out to me. I run faster.

And then, the now familiar blackout curtain falls, covering the rest of my night like a censor.

I see the stage. We are very far back. I fall backward.
I black out.

It's the end of the concert. I'm walking with the sea of people flooding down the stairs like water molecules to the exit. I am beside Emerson. I see a stranger with a very kind face. I have to tell him!
I black out.
(See Appendices P, Q.)

Kidnapped: Blacking Out, Dropping Names

I wake up without clothes on the top of a black bedspread.

Who is that!?

There's a guy, fully clothed, but in bed next to me. And another guy emerges in the doorframe shirtless. He has a kind face. He'll help me out. Wait! That's the guy with the kind face!

Meeting him on the stairs flashes in my mind.

"Let's go," the blonde guy in the doorway says.

"Huh? Who are you? Where am I?" I ask.

"You're at my house," the brunette guy in the bed says.

"Why?" I ask.

The boy in the doorway scratches his head, "I don't really know. You were drunk. Braden told me to take you with us," the kind-faced guy says and points to the clothed guy next to me.

Yeah, Braden looks like a dick.

I black out

I nudge Braden after getting dressed.

Of course, that's logical. Kidnap the drunk girl. Why hadn't Emerson stopped them?

"Can you take me home? I'm sorry…" I ask Braden.

"Sure. We've got to take Ian to the train anyway," Braden says.

"Who?" he points from under the comforter to the blonde guy who's just showed up in the doorframe again.

I guess the kind-faced man is named Ian.

"Where's Emerson?" I ask.

"Who?" Braden asks.

"The guy I was with," I answer.

"You were alone," Braden says.

Bullshit. No one goes to a concert alone.

"Nothing happened, right?" I ask.

"No way," Braden answers quickly.

"Nope," Ian says, "You wouldn't let us touch you. You were very good about that. But you did tell us you were a famous engineer and that you would be all over every track that hits number one this year."

"Oh yeah, and that your name is Kali Rae Wheeler and that we can look you up!" Braden says.

Oh my god, they know my NAME!!

I use fake names now because I am so protective of with whom I share things. After being so open for so many years while medicated, I kicked up enough dust to keep me coughing for the rest of my life. To clear things up a little bit, I plan on refusing to add to the conversation for the next few years, at least. I never want to leave a trace anymore. I want to be erasable: a phantom.

I sit in the backseat, behind Ian, the blonde guy. He is tall, probably six foot four. I find a half-drunk Gatorade and gulp it down.

I ask why I ended up at Braden's house and Ian explains that as they were leaving the concert, they saw me walking with Emerson.

They both assumed we were together, but I approached Ian and said, "You have such a kind face."

And I guess for them, that meant all bets were off, that I was a free woman.

This led to me going home with them, without my ride or friend and without any knowledge of where I was going.

While listening to the story, I thank God that these young men have a conscience. While I mull over and over the process of getting into their car and why, I also try to figure out why, if they'd kidnapped me, didn't they take advantage of me?

They had done everything else leading up to that point, but then they just let me walk. Taking me home with them alone is sketchy enough to fit the description of rapists.

Instead, they make fun of how "prudish" I acted while driving me home in the morning.

"Not even a little bit fun," Ian says.

And then I have a flashback to last night.

I come to, and find myself in Braden's bed. He is getting aggressive. Scared, I get up, searching for clues of where I am and looking for someone to help me get away.

I find "the kind face," Ian, sleeping on a mattress big enough for two. I climb in, fully clothed and explain to him I'm there to escape his friend, Braden, who is scaring me.

How could these random guys have been nice enough not to rape me and leave me to the wolves?

The brunette man doesn't seem like a nice person. He's self-centered, arrogant, and loves to describe his high-paying job, his designer labels and his new apartment with his seventy-inch plasma screen.

I want to barf.

"How did I meet you guys?" I ask.

"Wait, I thought you guys were friends from high school with Ian." Braden says, keeping his eyes on the road.

"What?!" Ian and I say in unison, me from the back seat, Ian riding passenger.

"No, I've never met him," I say.

Then it clicks.

The fact that Braden thought I was an old friend of Ian's saved me. Without that tiny bit of misunderstanding, I would probably have been taken advantage of and left out in the streets of that unfamiliar neighborhood. I would have had no idea where I was if it weren't for them driving me out of wherever we were.

My phone is sitting on the seat next to me: dead. Something must have happened with Emerson… He would have stepped in.

Right?

Is This a Home?

I come to.

There are three empty glasses in front of me, and one hardly touched brown drink. I am leaning on a marble bar.

Is this a hotel lounge or a home?

There are two men playing pool, another is making a drink behind the fully stocked bar, and a fourth, next to me at the bar. All of the men are in their mid-forties.

I recognize no one.

Where am I?

I get a flashback.

1. I am eating oysters with Avery.

2. We are drinking wine at his apartment in Hollywood. He sings "Slow Show" by the National and makes whiskey sours for both of us.

3. I'm getting out of an Uber and entering a club. Why, Kali?! NOOOOOoooooo.

4. I fight with Avery while drinking and as I slur my sentences as I am trying to explain. I recognize that I may be drunk. I get pissed and leave Avery, heading far into the center of the packed dance floor. I am lost in the crowd.

5. ...Nothing.

I try again.

6…Nothing.

All I have is that terrifying feeling when you know there is something your brain refuses to recall. It is the worst feeling.

What could have happened?

Avery and I enter the club together.

Why are we at the club? I hate clubs.

Anxiety rises, and I panic.

"Can someone take me home? Where is my phone?" I say and glance around the bar.

"I don't know," the guy next to me answers. "Check your purse."

"My purse! Where is my purse?" I say, suddenly aware that I have a purse that I don't currently have with me.

The powerful, stunning zap floods my body, and I'm dreading the inevitable.

"I put it in the guest room," another man answers.

"What? That's amazing. Where is that?" I ask exasperated.

"In there," he swings his pool cue to point at a small room across the dark living area. I run into the room.

My purse! My phone!

It's dead.

Dammit!

"Does anyone have a charger?" I ask while walking back toward the bar.

"No," a third guy says, half-listening.

"Okay, can somebody call me an Uber?" I ask.

"I'll take you," another man says.

"Can you take me now?" I ask, scared.

"No," he says.

"Okay. Well. Please don't leave without me. Please!" I say, oddly desperate. "No one has a charger?" I ask again.

"No," a couple of the guys respond in unison.

"Nope," the guy at the pool table adds.

I black out again.

It's Alright; A Woman Will Understand: NOT

I wake up naked, not entirely, but my bra is missing as well as my pants. I recognize the room and am brought back into my terrifying reality. I'm still at that mansion house.

I throw off the comforter and run into the living room where the bar is. At least I think this is a living room.

The early morning light shows that this must be some kind of den within the bigger house. This home is ridiculously big. I find my purse swung around a barstool. I find my phone again, still dead.

My wallet is gone. All that is in my purse are a couple of pieces of sandy Trident gum and a tampon.

I immediately grab my neck to check for my most-prized possession: the necklace.

It's not there.

"No! No! No! It couldn't have! It has to be here," I say.

I run back into the room and realize there's a man in the bed. I do not even recognize him from that group of five.

He is older. I wake him up aggressively.

"Please take me home! Where is my necklace? Please take me home, please, please," I shout. I'm crying now, "Who are you? Who are you?"

Over angry sobs I continue, "What happened? Where am I? I don't know where the fuck I am!" I buckle to the floor beside the bed, scared, but I continue yelling. I'm crying in the way you shout your tears out, choked by how angry you are, trying to muscle past the idea that you're crying.

"Who are you? What did you do? Please take me home. I'm begging you!" I scream.

I'm beyond devastated. I am lost and scared out of mind.

We could be anywhere in the world. This man could force me to be his sex-slave. He could kill me right there in his creepy mansion with his creepy friends. Or he could take me home.

"Go back to sleep," the man says.

"No!" I scream. "Get me out of here! I'm calling the cops!"

As soon as the idea hits that this place must have a landline, I run back out of the small room and into the living area.

"Sweetheart," he laughs standing in the doorway. "I'll take you in the morning. No one is looking for you."

"I need a phone," I say, realizing that I am trapped. I look back at him in the doorway, "Now!"

"Come back. I'll drive you in the morning," the man coaxes, motioning for me to come over to him.

FUCK THAT.

I take off running.

This place is huge!

Hallway after hallway of signed sports memorabilia and paintings.

Who is this guy? And why are there so many rooms?

I dash around the corners, nearly slamming into a sculpture on a pillar. There isn't one phone or anything in here that even looks lived-in … anywhere.

But, there are doors everywhere. I can hardly see straight. The immensity of the empty place isn't helping me grasp reality. I push on every door, one after the other. None are open! Not one!

Please, somebody!

I'm violently throwing myself into each door now.

Finally!

After what seems like the thirteenth door in this gigantic home, I stumble into an occupied room, falling onto the carpet.

"Help me! There's a man in your house! He took me here. I don't know where I am! Please, I just want to go home. Please help me!" I beg this person in this dark room. I can hardly see her form in the darkness of the room.

It's a small room, just a bed and a dresser, like a hotel. The woman on the bed pushes me away and I realize I had grabbed her shoulder in despair.

Her eyes are squinty. She's been asleep for a while.

Who is she? Is she that man's sister, a wife, friend?

Who cares?

A woman will understand.

"Get out of my room," the woman says.

"Please help me, please!" I grab the comforter, and the tears start flowing in confusion as she looks at me in anger.

"Get out of here!" she yells.

I leave the room, defeated, and run straight into the hairy chest of that man.

"Come back to bed. I won't touch you," the man says.

He puts his hands up like a criminal and then grabs my shoulders to reiterate.

I jump back, disgusted he thinks he can touch me like that. I am still without clothes, only a bra and underwear.

I'm completely helpless, and now hopeless in my search to get out of this underground trap. I feel like a dog being coaxed through the doors of the veterinarian's office.

I Swear I Won't Touch You

I follow the man back down the winding halls of perfectly groomed carpet. I am ready to endure whatever I have to endure. I want out with every piece of myself.

I can't believe she won't help me.

The man gets into bed after slipping off his sweats. I find my pants strewn in the corner, and put them on.

The shirtless, chain-wearing Persian man has his head perched on his hand. He turns toward me to watch me fumble with my jeans. I slip behind the door, covering my chest. He has a sheet around his waist.

Shit.

The necklace! I remember.

"You're so shy," he says with a smirk.

"Take me the FUCK home. I'll seriously hurt you if you try to touch me," I respond.

Great, Kali, make the kidnapper mad. Good plan.

He looks at me like he's going to smack me.

Stay strong, Kali.

I hold his gaze, staring directly into his pupils, building emotion inside me until I can feel the hormones surge through my body. The weight of past experiences and the knowledge that I am not alone in this fuels the fire.

I'm ready to attack.

After a couple of minutes, right as I am about to tear him the fuck up if he breathes in my direction, I watch his face soften. He transforms from predatory to angry.

Victory!

Whatever it is I have done, he gives up his pursuit.

"I swear I won't touch you," the man says.

He lies down, grabs the comforter and pulls it over himself, rolling over to face the other direction.

When he starts snoring, my body relaxes, allowing me to feel exhaustion taking over. A migraine snatches my eyesight, as I silently lay myself on top of the covers as far away from the man as possible without ending up on the dirty wood floor again.

The room spins.

"I'll take you back in the morning. Go to sleep," he groans.

Silence.

I move an inch more to the left so that my body is nearly off the bed entirely.

I pray someone rescues me.

Who was that girl?

Wendy's and a Business Card

An unintentional mind-travel transpires as the darkness behind my eyelids evolves into the beach in the film *Contact*.

My arms crossed over my body, like an angry mummy. I lie on top of the comforter, scared stiff, from about four a.m. on, eyes open, almost meditative, unblinking.

He wakes up and turns to face my direction. I'm standing by the bed.

"Where is my necklace?" I ask.

"I don't know. I didn't see a necklace," he says.

"It has a key on it. It is very special to me. Please help me find it," I say. I shovel all of the blankets off the man and off of the bed.

"Hey!" he shouts, angry.

I don't give a shit; this could not get worse. Now I just want my necklace. At least I'll be butchered with my necklace on.

I get back onto my hands and knees and I roam around in the darkness again, throwing the comforter up like a parachute as I continue the search.

"Hey, Kali," the man taunts having gotten out of bed to stand over me as I search.

"Fuck you," I say and don't look up at him. I continue crawling in the dark.

"Look what I have!" he says, dangling the necklace in front of me.

I snatch it in reflex, almost slicing his face with my nails by accident. I glare at him while dropping the comforter I'd thrown about in search of my prized possession.

"Thanks… Can you take me home now?" I ask.
I'm still unsure if he will ever take me home.
"Yes, ma'am," he says.
"Nothing happened, right?" I ask.
I'm shaking now that I realize I might live.
"No, you wouldn't allow it. You kept hitting me away," he says.
Yeah, then that would have been consensual, dude. Why for fuck's sake is there a "kept" and an "-ing" in that sentence?
Like, come on!

There are so many things wrong with how that night turns out.
I am so lucky that this man doesn't have his four friends gang bang me. He had to have known that if I were drunk enough to get in a strange car with five strange men, I was drunk enough to be raped and not remember the details enough to report it.

On the freeway home, he asks if I want to stop and get Wendy's.
"If you want to do that…" I say. I look at him with my best Puss in Boots eyes. "You'll still take me home, right?"
"Yes, of course, doll," the man says kindly.
"Okay, I'll do that, I'll get a burger," I say.
I'm pretty much incapable of life right now. So yeah, I'll eat a damn Wendy's burger, why the fuck not.

He buys me a burger and jokes the whole way to the apartment building about me never having tasted a Wendy's Burger.
As I exit his spotless black Tesla, he hands me his business card. I take it awkwardly. It says "Barry: owner."

"I own Brick and Oven. I don't know if you've heard of it—" Barry says.
"Uh, yeah, I think so. Awesome," I say.
It is a famous spot.
I've heard of it millions of times. Holding my heels in one hand and a Wendy's bag in the other, I stumble away from the car into a locked door to Avery's parking garage. Giving in to the shitty situation, I sit on the wall at the entrance to the garage. All I can do is wait.

My brain is so emotionally fried that I am not even aware of time. My mind is black, other than knowing how to chew the food in my mouth before I vomit up bile and whatever drug I was given last night.

I have zero intention of seeing or asking Avery what went down until I shower, sleep at my own apartment for at least eight hours, and any remnants of the terror of the night before have been swept under the rug by yours truly.

A couple leaving the apartment building's parking structure open the locked door for me in an act of pity.

I stumble in and beeline to my car.

Safety!

I can see the safe haven that is my Range Rover.

But not just yet.

"Kali! Kali!" Avery happens to be headed to his car AT THE EXACT TIME.

I look down, but I hear him shouting my name.

WHAT THE…

Fuck me.

I stop.

He rushes up to me, stopping only inches from my body.

"What are you doing?!" Avery says under his breath.

I keep my eyes on the ground.

"I just need to go home," I mumble.

What the…?" Avery says.

His voice is something I've never heard before. He gets even closer to me. I look up, and my eyes meet his, unintentionally.

His eyes are fixed on mine. His gaze like nothing I'd ever seen before: eyes-bulging, so angry. His hands are visibly shaking.

"Where did you go?" I ask.

"Where did I go?! You left me at the club! I turned around, and you're with these random dudes, and then you got in their car. How was I supposed—"

He reaches out and grabs my shirt. "This is inside-out. YOU SLEPT WITH SOMEONE!" he shouts and his voice echoes off the walls of the parking structure.

I look down to find my shirt, indeed, is inside-out.

Classy, Kali, real damn classy.

"What are you talking about. NO! He gave me pajamas," I lie and jump back.

I can't even try to explain the horror of what just happened, especially right now. I haven't even tried to look back on it yet. I'm still trying to take steps forward so that I am not raped and pillaged, or choke on my fries.

"Thank God he did," I continue to lie badly.

I try to explain that as much as Avery wants to believe I chose to get in that car, I simply did not. I don't even begin to explain how terrifying my night just was, and Avery doesn't ask. He is set on the fact that I bailed on him with five older men and therefore, stuck in his state of upset that I bailed on him.

HAHA.

A few days later, I have to go to Avery's to pick up a phone attachment I left while attaching my phone to his sound system. The things are expensive and I'm in school, so I pretend to be brave and head on over.

"I've just been through enough shit," I say.

"Go on..." he says.

"I've just experienced a lot of things, most of which I wish I hadn't," I reply.

"And..." Avery coaxes.

"And what? Stop asking me. I obviously don't want to talk to you about it," I say.

As he inquires further, I retreat faster. A few minutes later, I'm lacing up my combat boots to leave as he gives me an ultimatum.

"If you never let me know what you mean by shit, we will never get further than the surface. I don't want to be around you if you are not serious about opening up to me and moving forward," he says.

I smile sweetly and force my left foot into the other boot.

Why would I need to you tell you anything?

I never saw him again.

When Barry promises me he won't touch me, it rings so familiarly. Unfortunately, I have heard this same thing before, in other situations, in the same headspace.

When I drink, I don't want to be sexual. I am just overly friendly and adventurous. So if someone tells me that we should go to this party in the hills, and at the point of the asking I'm intoxicated, I'll probably agree wholeheartedly.

Aside from the many things I did wrong in this situation, well actually just one, drinking in the first place, this is one circumstance that still puzzles me.

I arrive at the club that night with a very tall, strong, award-winning actor. He is more than ten years older than me. His IMDB says he studied martial arts for twenty years and trained in multiple disciplines including; Brazilian Jiu-Jitsu, Muay Tai Kickboxing, Tae Kwon Do and hand-to-hand weapons combat. Avery is a model for video game heroes.

I am taken from the club, against my will (if I was conscious enough) by an out-of-shape, middle-aged asshole who probably couldn't hurt a fly if he wanted to hurt a fly.

How the hell did I get taken home by a group of random men when I had GI Joe as my date? (See Appendix P.)

Try: December 20, 2013,

I'm astonished
That as much as I may try
It all comes back to me full circle and I'm left right where I left off.

I want nothing
Because I've lost that ability

But I still have boundaries
So my circle keeps getting smaller,
And my eyes larger,
And yet the one thing that caught me off guard
Is the one thing I'll hold close to my heart
Because I wanted to feel something new
And I haven't felt anything since being with you,
Because nothing comes close to how it felt
And the words keep spilling out
But I've had nothing real to keep me full
So I play the same songs
And I dream the same dreams
And I never finished what I started
And I never finished what I started

Does it all reignite
Does it all get better
I've been stuck here for too long
I've been stuck here for too long
When you took me there
You never told me I'd have to find my way back
You showed me the view
But you didn't point out the land
So you helped me jump
But you didn't break my fall
It's like you opened my eyes to the darkness of the night
Because everything out up when I was with you
But you didn't let me know it was just temporary.

I ended up so lost
I shouldn't have taken so much
I ended up so lost
Searching for pages written somewhere

To lead me to the reason for all of this time
Why did I have to take an airplane to see you
Why did I have to go so far
You could have told me how simple this was
Before I took a dive into something so far gone
I wanted to stay
I did

But there were some things I had to finish
I wanted to leave it all behind
But there were things I couldn't decide on
and I wasn't sure you the one I could rely on
And so it's Christmas again
I didn't know it would come again this soon
Because the last time I truly felt alive
It was time for me to get on a plane to come see you
I still don't know
If it was only the drugs
I would think that if that was all
It was it would be easier to break this fall
It's been almost two years
And I've gone back in time
I've tried to relive our moments
But nothing, none of it even comes close to coming back alive.

Hungover at The Grammys: February 2013

"Okay! Can you guys tell me whose dressing room this one is?" the Grammy Foundation president asks the group.

"Rihanna for sure," a guy in our group says.

"Yes! We try to make their rooms as comfortable as possible. It can get pretty stressful. Too many creative minds in one place," the president says.

I feel like dying as we are led into the next artist's dressing room.

"Chris Brown!" a jerk yells.

I want to vomit, but instead, jam my fists farther into the front of the leather jacket. The one I'd found the last time I was in Toronto, the night Christina decided to disappear on us, leaving all of her things. She vanished for an entire day. Not contacting anyone, but leading me to have to call her parents, my parents and finally, the Canadian police. It was terribly unsafe for an American girl to be wandering around Toronto late at night.

Andriy's roommate, however, was throwing a party that night. So imagine how enthused everyone was when the police had to kick all of the drunk people out to take a statement from me.

Christina's bag was left unzipped. Everything from deodorant, to underwear, to her beat-up backpack, strewn everywhere. No sign of her.

I click back into the present.

"We use different signals for the mics; they are wireless, for obvious reasons. So it's very important to turn them off as the artist hands them to you coming off of the stage…" the man says.

I excuse myself to find the women's restroom and try and get my head in order.

When I rejoin the group, we are led to our seats. I finally get to sit and listen. Kelly Clarkson is unbelievably good and is also very sweet to the audio guy. Miguel is nervous and Mumford and Sons blows me away.

Of course, Taylor Swift doesn't rehearse. Her dancers are fabulous though, and remind me to take class in the morning as I recognize one of the dancers from class.

Maybe I'll just be a back-up dancer...

Aubrey

The event that Aubrey, my new boss, invited me to was definitely the highlight of my Grammy weekend. It was hosted by Quincy Jones and Al Schmitt. I'd met the pair several times and really enjoyed them. I didn't enjoy the hords of male music industry professionals, who I had met at previous music industry events, approaching me to offer me jobs that were actually just attempts to take me on a date.

After meeting a friend of Bill's at the TEC Awards, while acting as the usher to bring Paul McCartney and Slash to the podium to accept their awards, I get another dose of "pretend to care about your intellect, but I actually just want to get into your jeans." It is alright; I end up helping the guy work through the divorce his wife had recently filed after his own bandmate alerted his wife, with whom he shared three young, beautiful children with, that he'd slept with someone else.

It is awful to watch. When I first start working for him he has a beautiful office in downtown Los Angeles. By the end, we are moving his stuff into a loft in downtown Los Angeles. It will double as his office/studio *and* his home.

I help him purchase a comforter, set up his nightstands and offer comments like: "Yeah, I really do like this little closet. It's interesting and you definitely have a lot of light."

Aubrey comes over, looks into it. "I agree…" There's a long pause. "Have you seen a picture of the guy my wife is fucking?" It comes so out of nowhere and I spit the ginger tea he made for me all over the new hardwood floors. "Kali, he looks like Santa Claus, like fucking Santa Claus. I swear to you. My wife is fucking Santa." He's talking in his adorable, chronically hoarse voice, laughing, while scrolling through his iPhone. "I'm so serious…." Aubrey says.

He turns the phone around to reveal a man that actually *does* look *exactly* like Santa Claus.

4 Epilogue

Under the Lights: They're Chanting My Name

I peer around the edge of the curtain hanging in front of the second wing of the stage. The auditorium is full. I've only come here a handful of times to see my favorite bands play. Tessa even happens to work here as a bartender! (My best friend throughout middle and high school, for those who didn't read Book I yet…yet :).

I glance at the front row. The hardcore fans look my way and begin to chatter among themselves. They start chanting my name; some are being held back from the stage by security.

How did I make it here?

My Guide-Self answers without hesitation:

Well I know exactly how, by pushing and pushing and pushing and pushing and getting back up and trying again until no one, nothing could hold us back from becoming what we want to be: that's how.

I add a little "humph" at the end to show my dumb, cerebral-self it needs to wake up.

We did it, Kali. Because we never gave up.

My hair falls forward in front of me, and I realize that I am the only female in the prayer circle. I don't feel different. I wonder who'll do the prayer.

Bob begins. "Creator, thank you for this moment, and for the people that have come to this place to support what we are here to do…to the people on this team, let us all have health, wealth, and many more moments like this. In God's name, we pray. Amen."

"Amen," the group says in unison and breaks.

Only four of us now walk back up the steps to the wings. Now I am alone in the front wing.

The crowd begins chanting again.

The loud silence is deafening. When I stop moving for a moment, another wash of utter disbelief pumps my heart up to 150.

I don't even hear the crowd anymore. I am awash in gratitude and awe for everything that has happened up to now, to put me in the right place at the right time in magical, random organization.

The magnitude of the scope in which I have changed as a person from four years ago washes over me in waves. I am speechless.

Malik, the videographer, comes up behind me as the crowd begins to chant once more.

"I'll be right behind as you walk on," Malik says.

"Got it," I say.

I pace back and forth in the first wing, breathing and reciting affirmations. The crowd is so loud, no one can hear me.

I stand there motionless for a few moments, simply ready to perform: a tonic of sorts brewing within me.

Adrenaline surging as my nerves continue to run races around my body. It's a familiar feeling but not completely. In addition to the regular, excited nervousness I have felt before while standing on the starting blocks before a swim race, or watching in the wings as the house lights dim at my dance company's annual show, there is something new. Something I've been feeling every day, even while performing seemingly mundane activities. It is trust: trust in my Higher Self to perform: to conquer any problems that may arise.

My mind still wants to fight what my heart and body already know.

But you didn't sound check… Is the mic high enough?

The mic is the only outlier to the situation.

"You good?" Bob asks.

His face never changes, always calm confidence. It's like he's exhaling it to me.

"You got this," he repeats, in an even lower tone but not softer.

"You're gonna do great," I manage to say.

He doesn't respond to that, but rather repeats, "You got this," even more steady, "Have fun, Kali, just be you."

The song begins, I jump forward onto the stage and exhale before recalibrating my strut to center stage under the spotlight. Malik jumps out in front of me for a moment navigating his camera inches from my face. My boots hit the stage with a sound that means more to me than anything.

This is the end of my old story. This is the beginning of a new life, a divine life, co-created by yours truly in divine truth.

Because, as a good friend once told me:

"It's time now, Dear."

Afterword

The purpose of all of this painful recollection, reconciliation and research into my own past to piece together this forgotten mess, is to warn potential victims of any of the topics I cover. It is a call for action, a call to beam the spotlight on the darkest parts of our beautiful country in order to transcend to a healthier more peaceful, more loving population.

It is a gun pointed toward the Goliath companies and organizations that threaten to murder our children. It is a battle cry against the pharmaceutical companies profiting from people's misery and in the face of those who take advantage of others when they are not able to properly fight back.

It is a bomb ready to drop on the organization that shelters the criminals of these selfish acts of abuse.

This is a battle cry from a now twenty-something Indigo Child who cheated death to finally find herself enough, to warn the younger ones, by at least telling her story.

You are the light! You are special! You are SUPPOSED to shine brighter than everybody else. You are the New World Order. Stay safe because we've gotta turn steer this ship home to the right harbor.

Malik walked off stage with the Champagne he had just sprayed on the audience, and looking at the bottle I got a surge of anxiousness and remorse, the same feeling I had the day after the attack happened.

I felt a responsibility to say to the girls backstage: "I got sick drinking out of one of those once, so be careful."

And then to watch them and that bottle like a hawk to make sure they weren't drinking from it too frequently. I want to just put it in the trashcan, but that's not my decision to make. We only need one tribute for this situation. I've walked it; you don't need to walk there now.

Another night, another blank space, a stifling black hole.

Rather than a night that should have included texting my best friend, Tessa about dancing with my favorite singer, before falling asleep with my makeup on in my gorgeous apartment with my dog Stella, it's a memory of feeling worthless, guilty and that all too familiar, stomach-sickening terror of a dark night. An intense feeling of promising myself that I'd never, ever go back to that place in my mind, to find out what really went down while I was not conscious.

I have continued to write these books in the hope that someone might just stop and think before doing one of the things that took me to such a dark place. Maybe just for a moment save this person from themselves. I know it's tempting to experience something for yourself, but in the case of medications, you aren't experiencing anything; they are taking away your ability to experience precious moments in time.

Moving Forward, Battles & Being Alone

As I look through this timeline, I realize a few things. But the thing that stands out to me the most is how many crises were organized and fought. So many things went down in a span of three years, I have had enough action for the rest of my life. I was also never without a man by my side. Well, a boy, most of the time. But I always had someone going through these crises, if not causing them, holding my hand to find the way out or allowing me to drop theirs to find my own way out. There was always someone cheering me on.

Because I know so much so what it is like to have someone always there, I've really enjoyed the past year being completely alone. I do wish I had kept in contact with girlfriends from the past, but when you are going through this intense a transformation, it's a little tough for anybody to want to be a part of the ride, especially if they aren't receiving anything in the process.

I have spent the past year battling old mindsets and addictions and trying my best to overcome the crippling anxiety that I've always stored deep in the vaults of myself. I have come to face that nagging eating disorder once again, and I have learned how important it is to foster friendships and to listen. I have learned that I, alone, can do incredible things, and they don't always require incredible effort.

I was featured on every track of a number one album in America just simply because the artist liked talking to me and enjoyed the sound of my voice.

I can fix things and set up things. I can hook speakers up and cable and monitors for myself. I know which cables to buy at electronics stores and which buttons to press to turn things on. I know how to be self-sustaining.

And I've learned that no matter how beautiful you are, it doesn't matter if you don't feel beautiful. I've become more confident in my dealing with people and in my ability to efficiently communicate with others, and I have struggled on the other end with losing all my confidence when it comes to body image and physical attraction.

I have gained sixty pounds, if I go back to my pre-rehab weight, and I have now lost about twenty of that. I have found that I am fearful of men who pay me attention. I would rather not be seen when I am walking around the grocery store or to my job in Santa Monica, than be asked for my number. I have spent a good amount of time wishing I was completely invisible and covering myself up in every way possible without wearing a bag over my head. Pretty is something that I don't strive to be, sadly, I strive to look like I did before any of this went down.

I strive to be the budding teenager who was good at everything she tried and was labeled the "perfect" youngest child. I was small, athletic, cute and intelligent. And I had no baggage. I only know am realizing that what I strive to be is that eleven-year-old girl who hadn't been tricked and manipulated by this conniving world.

On another note, I have been protected. I have been thrown into situations most would not have survived, or at least would have come out of as a completely different person with a hardened soul. I am not very trusting. This is true. But I have not lost my kind heart in dealing with other people. I may be fearful and secretive at first, but I check myself to make sure I am not placing another person's past actions on this person's shoulders. This is a daily struggle and it is one I believe I will fight until the day I find solace and peace in someone other than my close family.

I have learned that emotions can be false. You can feel something that isn't true and you can feel it all the way down to the core of you. However, your intuition is something that you should treasure as your most valuable gift. Intuition is different from emotion. Emotion is in reaction to an event, and this has to do with the perception of how that even felt to you. Intuition is a gut feeling about something that you know is not right or you know is right.

In all of these years, it was when my intuition was jilted that I got myself into the scariest of situations with the darkest of individuals. My antenna was out and it was picking up on even the smallest of hints of sparkly pathways, *but,* it was bent and pinging me toward the wrong destination. It was this impulse control problem that allowed me to dart toward the way that was new and interesting. The idea that something could be more than what it seemed was just too enticing and to uncover a diamond in the rough was almost a fascination. I was set on proving the world wrong. And, in harnessing this Taurus behavior, I simply became the bull chasing the swinging red cloth.

I saw signs in everything that I did. I couldn't go a day without connecting one meeting to another. I had to see something in everything I did. And if it wasn't there, I would find it. Every moment had to have a purpose, but it's not like I started out with one necessarily. I made everything about something else that I had seen. I was pulling signs from previous, happier times and connecting them with graffiti I saw on a Dumpster or lyrics I heard from a street musician.

I lived in a place where my days were consumed with feeling that I should be doing something more important or more universal, but had no plan to bring it into fruition. I woke up early, I took my pills, I read, I played guitar, I cleaned, I organized, I found new health essentials and then I worried. I worried and worried and worried and worried that I needed a sign to show me where to turn next.

At this point, I've only started to realize that you put yourself into motion and things start happening. You might not know the destination, and the destination might be a completely different highway to a completely different town, but you have to be in this spot in this piece of time and space to construct the building block for the next part of the journey.

Now more than I ever, I see dreams that I vaguely had for myself coming true, not in the time period I had allotted or in the way I had imagined, but they are happening. Flexibility has been a blessing. And I realize that the way I plan things to happen will most likely not be how they do happen. Sometimes, though, when looking through a different lens, I am able to see that they did happen in the way I thought they would. Living for each day, rather than for tomorrow, and gratitude.

There is also as much finality in an event or chapter of your life, that you allow there to be. There are holes that I still keep open, partially subconsciously, so that I am able to work through them in the right time and in the right mind. Possibly, I need to keep those wounds open so that they can heal after I am through with the process of reliving them for the book. I have completely shut the door on several people and have no emotions toward them but indifference and pity. Others I keep in my heart so treasured I'm not sure I'll ever have the ability to explain it to them in the correct fashion without them thinking that I'm in love with them or want to go back to a time when I was, we were, together.

There are still some people that pain me to think about. Most times due to the fact that they tried so hard to pull me back out of this sort of coma I was in and I was unresponsive. They tried and tried and ultimately gave up. I pulled them too hard one way with no give. It's the people who tried to pull the real person out of the costume that have pieces of my heart with them today. It's those people who saw two sides of this picture. They saw the unmedicated Kali and the medicated Kali and didn't understand why I chose the second or felt I needed to choose the second. The ones who didn't manipulate the situation or feel that they could put one over on me or minimize me until I felt unworthy of anybody but themselves.

I see now that the opportunistic people were just fearful. They were afraid I would see the real person hiding behind their caretaker persona. It was so easy for them to see that I'd wake up one day and realize I didn't need them around and once more, I didn't want them around! They were scared that I'd realize I didn't need their help, guidance or any of the meds that made it seem okay to talk down to me. They didn't want that comfort taken away from them so that they couldn't ask out of context questions while in a serious argument about drug-use, abuse or cheating, if I'd taken my meds.

Stealing My Adolescence

It's not all the time that you can say a situation had a specific starting point and a specific ending point. In this case, the ending point seemed to be all too eager right from the start. The starting point was a simple yet potent misdiagnosis of a hypersensitive teenager who wanted a reason for why she felt different. The ending was the realization that this was all self-made. A diagnosis was an alibi to help with the difficult times.

Western medical doctors are trained in Western medicine, which, in this day and age, is run by the pharmaceutical companies. If you are trained to find illness and treat said illness with medicine, a patient can logically assume if they come to see you, you will find something that needs to be treated with medicine.

In our society we view doctors almost as gods. They are put on a pedestal. We are conditioned to trust them and tell them all of the things we don't dare tell another soul. We literally entrust them with our lives. We put the responsibility for our health upon our physicians. We put full trust in this product, the doctor.

If your doctor is pure in his intentions, holding no belief systems that would influence his or her diagnosis, having no restrictions or if so, stating them out loud to you, on his practice, and eager enough to learn each and every day he puts on that white coat, as well as, an impenetrable shield against stressors, outside influence, stereotypes and bribes, you're in a pretty good place when it comes to trusting him with your life.

But still then, you and only you hold the responsibility for your health, your life. You are the only person who cares enough to find the answers to the questions that have never been asked, forget answered.

Most of us don't have God as our family physician. Actually most of us don't even see our doctors for more than the fifteen minutes allotted tby the insurance providers.

This system has the ability to ruin lives. I was able to see from the outside in because of my relationship with my family, and due to my faith in a higher power. I drew people into my life who understood that I was taken captive by medicines and diagnoses that just didn't fit the person that I truly was inside. Boyfriend after boyfriend told me they liked me better when I hadn't taken my medications. It took way too many of those painfully and mistakenly honest expressions on people's faces.

It took way too many different therapists and medical doctors and way too many tests and hospital visits, to come to the conclusion that this was all self-made. Can somebody really think themselves into a state of complete and utter devastation and then talk each of these medical doctors into seeing the difficult reality I was experiencing?

Did they know that I was simply an oversensitive, overly intelligent young girl who wasn't going to be satisfied without an answer, so they made the decision to make one up? Did I not fit into their minds in the neat categories that they were trained to compartmentalize their patients in. Is this why my entire adolescence and young adulthood was taken from me?

Having No Interest in Drugs or Alcohol

It's interesting that once I stopped the medications that were messing with my neurotransmitters, the ones that I had been on since I was in middle school, different ones for different made-up reasons, I have zero interest in alcohol or drugs.

Two years after stopping the last medication, Depakote, in 2013, I found that it had been about a year since I drank anything. And prior to that one night about a year ago, it had been months since my last drink and that night didn't end well.

After reading up about the effects of manipulating neurotransmitters and parts of the brain that regulate your impulses, addictions and ability to appropriately judge and respond to different situations, it seems that the drugs I was on not only lit up the stress response in my brain, but turned off the neurotransmitters that would say "STOP!" They also released more of the neurotransmitters that said "GO!" and then turned off everything when there was too much, leading to blackouts.

I will probably never know, but I wonder daily due to my complete aversion to even tasting alcohol when it is mixed into herbal remedies, and my mother's lifelong aversion to the smell and taste of alcohol as well, if the entire span of drinking so much and getting into opiates stemmed from the positive reinforcement chemicals lighting up my brain from the meds.

I will never know. But I will always wonder.

I never looked forward to the taste of alcohol. It was only once I had gotten down the first few shots and the haze came over me that I could keep drinking. By then, I couldn't taste anything or feel my headache; I just wanted to escape.

And anyone around me at the time would say I acted completely normal but drank more alcohol than they would ever imagine I could or even did. (See Appendices O, K, P, N.)

The years of my life that I can't remember or incidents that I have to have retold to me from times when I had not had anything to drink but just don't remember, seem like they were run from an entirely different brain than the one I was born with and the one I have now.

It is overwhelming daily. And I am so grateful to have found myself again after so many years of wanting so badly to feel alive.

I have not been suicidal, manic, or depressed since stopping those medications years ago. I have my days and feel that I might have to work harder then some to find peace. But I understand my duty to be here and to live each day as if it is my last, understanding that it could be. And many times, it should.

On Life as a Task

Life becomes easier when it all boils down to a task, something that can be aided and fixed with easy to grab tools. That's the thing though; life is not an everyday task. It is not simply a task; it is something that you have to learn to manage, not just get through unscratched with a checkmark.

Life isn't about checkmarks and it's also not about finding a solution when you don't feel perfect. Actually most of the time you won't feel perfect. That's what allows change to take place. Most of the time you will have to change what you are doing in order to get different results, not change what medicines you are taking.

APPENDICES

APPENDIX A

RX FX: DEXEDRINE (DEXTROAMPHETAMINE SULFATE)

Within days of starting to take this drug, I total my Range Rover in Malibu on Pacific Coast Highway on the way to a photoshoot.

Under the Warnings section of the drug labeling, the following conditions are listed:

> Amphetamines may impair the ability of the patient to engage in potentially hazardous activities such as operating machinery or vehicles; the patient should therefore be cautioned accordingly (The Food and drug Administration [FDA]).'

I wasn't warned about driving, since I drove to that appointment and drove back with a prescription for a stimulant and zero instructions.

Also, a new black box warning on Dexedrine warns that children and adolescents [under the age of 24] are at risk for sudden death (Medscape 2016).

These are side effects listed on the medication guide.

All Patients

- new or worse behavior and thought problems
- new or worse bipolar illness
- new or worse aggressive behavior or hostility:

Children and Teenagers

- new psychotic symptoms (such as hearing voices, believing things that are not true, are suspicious)
- new manic symptoms

APPENDIX B

RX FX: DEPAKOTE (DIVALPROEX SODIUM)

> BLACK BOX FOR BIRTH DEFECTS
> BLACK BOX FOR POTENTIALLY DEADLY PANCREATITIS
> BLACK BOX FOR POTENTIALLY DEADLY HEPATOXICITY***

PART A. COMING TO

Depakote is the last psychotropic drug I ever took. I can't pinpoint the moment it all came rushing over me, this wave of knowing that I *wasn't* sick. All through my happy childhood I didn't have an issue. I'd always been more thoughtful than others.

I wrote pretty intense poetry in elementary school and could hold significant conversations with adults, but I wasn't ever bipolar.

"You were polar sometimes, yeah," my mom says, "But before they woman gave you Prozac you were never manic."

I noticed my hair getting significantly thinner and I would have gruesome hangovers. Hangovers that had me laid-out, on my back, all day, no matter whose place I had been at the night before.

I'd spend the day sweating, crying, vomiting, and feeling like I didn't have the strength to press down the cap to my Synthroid medication.

I was at a fellow audio engineer's home in the valley when I woke up to a very tall geode. I looked around the room and saw three more and just as I was beginning to think I had woken up in heaven.

Christian walks into the room with a leopard cat. He asks. "You having that reaction again?"

He sets water next to the bed. "The one to that seizure medication you take?"

"Yeah, I can't move. Like, at all," I say.

Christian shakes his head, silky dirty-blonde hair putting my now dreadlocked fine brown hair to shame. From Christian's appearance, it is pretty obvious his mother was a famous model.

Christian is gorgeous, perfect body too. He turns to face the door and flings himself onto the bed, unannounced and nonchalantly. We've only

---

*** drug-induced liver damage that may lead to liver failure and death (Abbot 2017)

hung out to write music a couple times and I didn't plan on waking up in this heaven of a room: The floor is all wood, the light brown kind, and the duvet is crisp white. I've never felt a more comfortable mattress and the fluff from the pillow is engulfing me. The mattress is firm enough to support my lolling head, which feels even more heavy than usual. I can't flinch to move away, so I shove away any restrictions on body proximity and simply let it be.

Christian is strictly a friend, but the ease of his personality with me is magnetic. He is light.

"Kali, have you ever even *had* a seizure?" Christian asks.

"No," I say.

"Why do you take an anti-seizure medication then?" he says.

"Well…I got—" I start, but my subconscious shouts at me to stop trying to defend myself. "I don't know."

"You should go to my doctor," Christian says fumbling with a lock of his own hair, and staring up at the light above the bed. He turns his head to look at me.

God dammit.

"Kali?" Christians says, staring at me through brown, doe eyes. He looks like a doll, perfectly tan, chiseled jawbone, eyelashes I envy.

"Yes Christian," I say. I prepare for something awkward and wrack my brain for reasons why the hell I thought coming to the valley last night to work on my project was a good idea. He does play piano really well. I needed keys on that track.

"You're in my little sister's bed," he says and laughs like a little boy at his nailed attempt to make me feel like he was about to say something weird.

I laugh until my ribs hurt. I put my arms up to shield myself from the light above me, realizing it's giving me a migraine.

"Yeah, that's a problem for sure," Christian says and grabs a t-shirt out of the wooden dresser next to the bed and throws it over the top of the elegant, glass fixture.

When the dust settled, and I'd been out on my own for a few years, moving to the valley (somewhere none of my family members understood, along with my affinity to work in the audio world) and saw Christian's mother's doctor, who in fact was and still is a magical genius wizard man, I realized that Depakote was doing nothing for me. There wasn't any sort of reason to start taking it. I shuffled through so many psychiatrists and behavioral/mental health therapists in college that I actually lost track of the doctor who had originally prescribed me this medicine.

Dr. B advised me to stop taking it in a long dissent and I did. I don't remember much of it, except that the terrible hangovers subsided and my hair started growing back.

PART B. FINED BY THE FDA, MISLEADING ADVERTISING

The company that makes Depakote also illegally marketed the drug. It is an anti-seizure medication, FDA approved to treat bipolar disorder and migraines, but…

> Its manufacturer Abbott settled a case for $3 million in Arkansas for illegally promoting it to treat schizophrenia and autism, and it settled a $1.5 billion case for illegally promoting it to elderly dementia patients (Drugwatch 2017).

A letter was written to the Food and Drug Administration [FDA] addressing the concerns about Depakote's serious side effects. Not only is it a dangerous drug without marketing, Abbot laboratories, the makers of Depakote were forced by the FDA to correct false and misleading advertisements for the products. The statements in the advertisement omitted risk factors, added benefits, and overall, misled the consumer into thinking Depakote ER did something more than its predecessor, Depakote.

> …it implies that Depakote ER is indicated for use in a broader range of mania patients than Depakote, when this is not the case. Specifically, the Flashcard includes the following claim (emphasis added): "Expanded acute mania indication with Depakote ER that includes mixed episodes associated with bipolar disorder, with or without psychotic features"
> This statement misleadingly suggests that Depakote ER is indicated for a broader mania population than Depakote. In fact, the populations studied in the mania clinical trials of both products were selected using a broad interpretation of acute mania in bipolar disorder, and as described in the Pis for both products, there were no clinical differences between the mania populations studied for each drug (Toscano 2017).

PART C. ANTI-EPILEPTIC TO BIPOLAR TREATMENT TO MIGRAINE TREATMENT

> More than two million Americans have some form of epilepsy, and 125,000 new cases of epilepsy are reported each year. For the drug maker, Abbott Laboratories, sales

were brisk, but there were other markets to tap into - also known as "off-label" use (Mundy 2017).

Since being approved for the off-label use of treating manic episodes in patients suffering from bipolar disorder, Depakote has become the most-prescribed drug for manic depression. Lithium had been the only FDA-approved medication for mania up until the introduction of Abbott Laboratories' Depakote. Only a year after the introduction of Depakote for the use in manic depression, Depakote was approved by the FDA as a migraine treatment.

> The drug company maximized Depakote by advising migraine patients to take the medication "daily to reduce the frequency of migraine headaches," said Andre Pernet, Ph.D., vice president, pharmaceutical research and development, Abbott Laboratories.

Four years after Depakote's introduction into the manic depressive scene…

> …reports of life-threatening pancreatitis, the FDA required black box warning … In a recent letter, Abbott describes some of the cases as hemorrhagic with a rapid progression from initial symptoms to death (Mundy 2017).

Another seven years later,

> The FDA approved further safety labeling revisions to advise of the risk for congenital malformations in infants exposed to Depakote during gestation … animal studies have shown an adverse effect … (Mundy 2017).

PART D. HOW DOES DEPAKOTE WORK? WHY SO MANY USES?

> The active ingredient in Depakote is divalproex sodium. It works to increase levels of the brain neurotransmitter gamma aminobutyric acid (GABA). GABA's function in the body is to carry brain cell messages and soothe overstimulated nerves. This soothing quality makes Depakote a suitable treatment for epilepsy… Depakote increases GABA, which helps to prevent these electrical changes (Drug Dangers 2017). (See Appendices M, O, P.)

PART D. DEPAKOTE WITHDRAWAL

One of the most significant and most common antipsychotic withdrawal side effects is having a seizure, even if you take this anticonvulsant medication for bipolar disorder or migraines and have never previously had a seizure; there is the risk of having a seizure while coming off Depakote. These seizures may be very serious, severe, and potentially very hard to control. Other severe withdrawal symptoms include extreme bipolar episodes and excruciating migraines (Alternative 2017).

APPENDIX C

RX FX: XANAX (ALPRAZOLAM)

I found the black box warning labeled "Use with Other CNS Depressants" particularly frightening:

> The benzodiazepines, including alprazolam (Xanax) produce additive CNS depressant effects when coadministered with other psychotropic medications, anticonvulsants, antihistaminics, ethanol and other drugs which themselves produce CNS depression (Drugs.com 2016).

APPENDIX D

RX FX: VYVANSE AND ADDERALL

PART A. $56.5-MILLION VIOLATION OF THE FALSE CLAIMS ACT

> Shire Pharmaceuticals LLC will pay $56.5-million to
> resolve civil allegations … as a result of its marketing and
> promotion of several drugs, [Vyvanse, Aderall XR,
> Dayrana] the Justice Department announced today. … The
> settlement resolves allegations that, between January 2004
> and December 2007, Shire promoted Adderall XR for for
> certain uses … based on unsupported claims that Adderall
> XR would prevent poor academic performance, loss of
> employment, criminal behavior, traffic accidents and
> sexually transmitted disease. (DOJ 2017).

In addition, Shire allegedly promoted Adderall XR for the treatment of
conduct disorder.

PART B. MISLEADING STATEMENTS ABOUT EFFICACY AND ABUSEABILITY

> The settlement further resolves allegations that, between
> February 2007 and September 2010, Shire sales
> representatives and other agents allegedly made false and
> misleading statements about the efficacy and 'abuseability'
> of Vyvanse to state Medicaid formulary committees and to
> individual physicians … (DOJ 2017).

APPENDIX E

RX FX: TOPAMAX (TOPIRAMATE)

REQUIRES BLACK BOX ON SUICIDALITY

PART A. KIDNEY STONES

For me, Topamax, or "Dopamax" (Smyres 2017) lives up to its name. Along with the immense word-finding difficulties that I ironically "can't seem to pinpoint or describe" (see *Book I: Losing Kali* and *Book II: Missing Kali* for more.) Topamax stars in a handful of late-night trips to the emergency room.

The "doping" symptoms I describe in Books I and II fall away within months. The kidney stones formed during the year or so on Topamax are a whole different story, literally.

Kidney stones don't just evaporate. They don't just go away; you have to pass kidney stones. You pee out tiny rocks. I peed out a couple dozen of these small rocks over a two-year period and visited multiple specialists who diagnosed me with interstitial cystitis and prescribed me Macrobid and Detrol LA.

"Treatment with topiramate causes systemic metabolic acidosis, markedly lower urinary citrate excretion, and increased urinary pH. These changes increase the propensity to form calcium phosphate stones" (Welch 2006).

Researchers at University of Texas Southwestern Medical Center also found, "Topamax; a drug commonly prescribed to treat seizures and migraine headaches, can increase the propensity of calcium phosphate kidney stones" (UT Southwestern Medical Center 2006).

And, just in case you needed more proof for the emergency room visits, years after I stopped taking Topamax, at the National Kidney Foundation 2013 Spring Clinical Meetings, Allan Jhagroo, MD, an assistant professor of medicine, presented his study:

> Patients who take topiramate (Topamax) therapy for treatment of migraine appear to deplete citrate in the urine, creating an environment for kidney stones, researchers reported here. Within 30 days of the onset of topiramate therapy, mean urinary citrate excretion decreased 279 mg a day… Hypocitraturia from topiramate is rapid and progressive. What surprised us, was that at 60 days the

reduction in citrate output continued to progress (Susman 2013).

Jhagroo's team of researchers noted: "that at 60 days, six of the seven patients … hypocitraturic, with a mean 196 mg/day of urinary citrate excretion … citrate excretion of less than 320 mg a day clearly puts patients at risk for stone development … None of these patients had a history of kidney stones…" (Susman 2013). Program chair, Charmaine E. Lok, MD, medical director of the Renal Management and Hemodialysis Vascular Access programs at the University Health Network at Toronto General Hospital told *Medpage*:

> Silence is a key feature in many aspects of kidney disorders; as such, there needs to be a greater awareness of the largely asymptomatic chronic kidney disease that affects approximately 13% of the U.S. population. However, one kidney disorder that can present quite dramatically is nephrolithiasis (kidney stones). Passing a kidney stone can be quite painful and unforgettable (Susman 2013).

PART B. DOPAMAX

This article seems to sum things up way better than I ever could while taking Topamax. Also, I was prescribed Topamax to treat the drug-induced bipolar disorder, but was told it would clear up my headaches too. (See Part C for more on this).

> Migraine preventive Topamax (topiramate) has long been associated with trouble thinking, hence the widely used nickname of Dopamax. A recent study indicates that some people have trouble with language while taking Topamax. Some 'language disturbances,' as the authors call it, include:
>
> - Finding words
> - Substituting a word with another unrelated word
> - Taking forever to get a thought out
> - Meshing words
> - Naming objects (Symres 2016).

PART C. SUICIDALITY

Topamax is a member of the antiepileptic class of drugs that causes an increase in suicidality (The Food and Drug Administration [FDA] 2009).

PART D. OFF-BRAND MARKETING LAWSUIT

To top it all off:

> The manufacturer, two subsidiaries of health care giant Johnson & Johnson, were found guilty of marketing the drug [Topamax] for unapproved treatments, such as weight loss and bipolar disorder. The Department of Justice fined Ortho-McNeil Pharmaceutical and Ortho-McNeil-Janssen Pharmaceuticals more than $81 million in 2010 for this dangerous practice (Drugwatch 2016).

APPENDIX F

RX FX: AVELOX, CIPRO, LEVAQUIN, FACTIVE (FLUOROQUINOLONES)

I got used to feeling bad. Whether it was from starving, medication reactions, or actual illness, I expected to feel loopy, headachy and nauseated. So when I was prescribed antibiotics, especially the big, white Cipro pill, I knew I'd be sick with the same symptoms until I was finished taking them.

Turns out, just this May, a serious FDA Black Box Warning was placed on not only Cipro, but on all fluoroquinolone antibiotics. I knew that a couple of these antibiotics caused everything from hallucinations to night terrors and paranoia in myself. I believed Cipro was a safe one.

Wrong again!

> The U.S. Food and Drug Administration (FDA) approved changes to the labels of fluoroquinolone. These medicines are associated with disabling and potentially permanent side effects of the tendons, muscles, joints, nerves, and central nervous system that can occur together in the same patient. As a result, we revised the boxed warning, FDA's strongest warning, to address these serious safety issues. We also added a new warning and updated other parts of the drug label, including the patient Medication Guide. Patients must contact your health care professional immediately if you experience any serious side effects while taking your fluoroquinolone medicine. Some signs and symptoms of serious side effects include unusual joint or tendon pain, muscle weakness, a 'pins and needles' tingling or pricking sensation, numbness in the arms or legs, confusion, and hallucinations (FDA 2016).

A few months later, a new statement was released, advising doctors to stay away from prescribing these drugs at all "because the risk of these serious side effects generally outweighs the benefits for patients." (FDA 2016) The reasons for prescribing these drugs include anthrax and plague.

> Because the risk of these serious side effects generally outweighs the benefits for patients with acute bacterial sinusitis, acute exacerbation of chronic bronchitis and

uncomplicated urinary tract infections, the FDA has determined that fluoroquinolones should be reserved for use in patients with these conditions who have no alternative treatment options. For some serious bacterial infections, including anthrax, plague and bacterial pneumonia among others, the benefits of fluoroquinolones outweigh the risks and it is appropriate for them to remain available as a therapeutic option. (FDA 2016).

After seven years, on July 25, 2016, the FDA approved the addition of a black box warning for a group of FDA-approved antibiotics (the most commonly prescribed antibiotic in the country) fluoroquinolones. These include; levofloxacin (Levaquin), ciprofloxacin (Cipro), moxifloxacin (Avelox), ofloxacin and gemifloxacin (Factive). (Llamas 2016)

The labeling changes include an updated boxed warning and revisions to the Warnings and Precautions section of the label about the risk of disabling and potentially irreversible adverse reactions that can occur together (FDA 2017).

This is all well and good. I'm glad there was movement in regard to the study. However, check out how long it took for just a label to be slapped on the medication manual:

- 2008: FDA puts first black box warning on fluoroquinolones for risk of tendinitis and tendon rupture.
- 2011: The risk of worsening symptoms for those with myasthenia gravis was added.
- 2013: Updated label with "irreversible peripheral neuropathy (serious nerve damage."
- 2015: An FDA advisory committee focused on two or more side effects occurring at the same time and causing the potential for irreversible impairment. The advisory committee concluded that the serious risks generally outweighed the benefits…
- July 26, 2016 The FDA approves label changes to enhance warnings about disabling and potentially permanent side effects and to limit use (FDA 2016).

It took them seven years! And this is the most commonly prescribed type of antibiotic! Seven years was enough time for me to lose my entire young adult and college life, in a trance due to a false diagnosis of symptoms triggered by prescription drugs. Seven years is way too long for 2016. We must change this before it ruins what we have left of the delicate fabric that is humanity.

APPENDIX G

BLACK BOX WARNING FOR ANTIEPILEPTIC DRUGS
[from Books 1 & 2]

Like their predecessors, the SSRIs, anticonvulsant drugs all got slapped with a black box warning for suicidality after studies were consistent across the board on eleven different drugs that these medications produce suicidal thoughts.

> AED class label changes: Manufacturers of antiepileptic drugs (AEDs) or anticonvulsant drugs will update product labeling to include a warning about an increased risk of suicidal thoughts or actions and will develop a Medication Guide to help patients understand this risk (FDA 2009).

The AEDs affected are listed below.

> Carbatro, Celontin, Depakene, Depakote ER, Depakote sprinkles, Depakote tablets, Dilantin, Equetro, Felbatol, Gabitril, Keppra, Keppra XR, Klonopin, Lamictal, Lyrica, Mysoline, Neurontin, Peganone, Stavzor, Tegretol, Tegretol, XR, Topamax, Tranxene, Tridione, Trileptal, Zarontin, Zonegran (FDA 2009).

Some of the signs of this suicidal behavior include:

- Talking or thinking about wanting to hurt yourself or end your life.
- Becoming preoccupied with death and dying.
- Becoming depressed or having your depression get worse.
- Withdrawing from friends and family.
- Giving away prized possessions (FDA 2016).

APPENDIX H

POST TRAUMATIC STRESS DISORDER

> Though only 10 percent of American forces see combat, the U.S. military now has the highest rate of post-traumatic stress disorder in its history…(Junger 2017.)

A female sufferer who since has recovered from PTSD does a good job at explaining what our body does when it is in constant fear and why:

> From an evolutionary perspective, it's exactly the response you want to have when your life is in danger: you want to be vigilant, you want to react to strange noises, you want to sleep lightly and wake easily, you want to have flashbacks that remind you of the danger, and you want to be, by turns, anxious and depressed. Anxiety keeps you ready to fight, and depression keeps you from being too active and putting yourself at greater risk. (Junger 2017.)

I know that in my life this particular aspect has played a starring role in the chaos, from flashbacks to nightmares to constant fear of overstepping my boundaries, or of someone finding me attractive.

However, I am nonetheless a strong woman, who perseveres as a victor and not a victim. And although it is something I refuse to accept sometimes, I say mantras multiple times daily in regard to not feeling guilty or worthless or worthy of terrible things. I constantly find myself thinking back to situations I should have seen coming or people I should have known were bad. I did this for so many years that I actually forgot who I was and still, today, have to remind myself that it is okay to draw attention or to have success or to feel good! It is also okay to show my legs and to wear a swimsuit and to play!

This is something that so many people are facing and trying to navigate themselves. You are not alone.

Sexual abuse is not something that happens to a certain type of personal with a certain type of personality or clothing or name; it happens to people from every background and every walk of life. And, it is spreading like wildfire in out culture. The fire is fed by systems in place that DO NOT help the victims but instead cause them to feel guilt, shame and remorse for telling someone. We have got to fix the issue of assault on college campuses. #ITSONUS

Also, today I was thinking about this particular book and trying to pick my memory for male teachers or leaders outside of my family that I could trust. And what I came up with was an insanely deep gratitude for the men of the audio engineering school I attended.

Not only were all of the professors helpful, extremely educated and polite, they never ONCE made me feel uncomfortable. None of the students did either. In fact, I was treated like a queen when I came to the recording studio after breaking my ankle. (The downstairs area of the college was lined with recording studios to practice in.)

The teacher set up a chair in the very center of the console for me to sit down instead of standing through the lecture. Those were true gentlemen. They even made sure I had someone to walk me around the corner to my car at night. Which, at this point in my life, made my heart sing. Every time it was offered, my heart was filled with hope that maybe not everyone wants to take something from me.

> Rape is one of the most psychologically devastating things that can happen to a person, for example—far more traumatizing than most military deployments—and, according to a 1992 study published in the Journal of Traumatic Stress, 94 percent of rape survivors exhibit signs of extreme trauma immediately afterward. (Junger 2017).

APPENDIX I

SEROTONIN SYNDROME AND PTSD

The thing about Serotonin Syndrome is it causes you to partake in risky behavior, or to even seek out dangerous situations. The problem here is that kids are being put on SSRIs, as I was in book one, switched around to different medications, all while trying to grow up and deal with high school and any kind of social life.

When you mix a brain filled with hormones, a developing brain, and psychotropic drugs, it is not going to end well most times, unless you are the person who was born with an imbalance. In this case, there should be careful instructions regarding alcohol use and the drug you are prescribed, as well as any other possible adverse reactions.

I was put on Prozac, and immediately jumped into an extremely bumpy ride of medication highs and lows, medication withdrawals and then into recreational pills to feel better. I was drinking in high school, although I stopped several times, I blacked out each time I drank. This went on through college.

Putting yourself in dangerous situations, a sign of serotonin syndrome, a syndrome brought on by an increase of serotonin in the brain usually in result of a medication switch or addition dealing with these chemicals but can also be brought on by ADHD meds, opiates and alcohol, leads to a breeding ground of PTSD origins.

Years later I found myself withdrawing from everyone. I gained weight in an attempt to protect myself. I shut everyone out, making sure that no more of me was revealed to the world. I felt I needed to scrub every asset of my life clean.

Although I tried, this desperate attempt at erasing my prior self, was to no avail. And I ended up bringing my messed up brain into new relationships and situations.

The medications I was given in high school continue to affect me to this day. I've not only lost people I love, but opportunities I truly feel are not as accessible to me because I lost the confidence to believe that anything good could be given to me or that I could be worthy.

I never once thought that I wasn't to blame for the rapes, for the car accidents, for the emergency room visits or the abusive boyfriends. I never even thought of it. I was engulfed in shame. And I work to this day on digging my way out of the guilt and shame that try to wreak havoc.

When I asked my parents tonight if they knew what Post Traumatic Stress Disorder was my dad replied promptly, "It is a disorder that is brought on by extreme trauma, like war or rape. It causes nightmares, stress, anxiety, inability to form and keep relationships, random crying, headaches…..."

My mom added, "It causes anxiety, flashbacks, stress…so much."

About an hour later, after a refreshing walk at the beach I asked them both a new question. "Do you guys know what Serotonin Syndrome is?" I said.

"Nope," my well-informed father said.

"I know from you. I know because you told me about it," my mom said.

APPENDIX J

POSTTRAUMATIC STRESS DISORDER [PTSD] AND MDMA

> About 8% of the US population will experience PTSD at some point in their lives. And up to half of participants enrolled in clinical trials to treat PTSD fail to respond to therapies including serotonin-reuptake inhibitors — a class of drugs often used as antidepressants — and cognitive behavioral therapy (Junger 2017).

PART A. MDMA TO TREAT PTSD

In the 1970s MDMA was experimented with by therapists and researchers. In the '80s the use became more recreationally used. By 1986, after years of hearings, a judge recommended MDMA be classified as a Schedule III drug, yet the DEA slapped it with a Schedule I label, deterring its use in therapeutic settings.

> [The judge] made three basic findings: that MDMA had a low potential for abuse; that it had an accepted medical use; that there was an acceptable level of safety for use under medical supervision.

In other countries, MDMA is already being used and with great success:

> They have used it to help individuals uncover painful childhood memories and experiences that had been repressed; to decrease fear and defensiveness; to increase communication and empathy with one's spouse; to get through traumatic experiences such as rape and incest; to live with the pain of cancer; and to resolve oneself to dying (Scharff 2017).

In a 2010 study where MDMA-assisted psychotherapy was compared with psychotherapy alone yielded tremendous results.

> 83% of PTSD patients treated with MDMA-assisted psychotherapy showed marked improvement, compared to 25% of those treated with psychotherapy alone. A follow-up study found that the majority of those treated with the

assistance of MDMA remained symptom-free two years later (Scharff 2017).

Just recently, at a conference in Oakland, California, the trial treatment that Dr. Mithoefer recommended, MDMA and psychotherapy, was moved forward into phase three, the last step before potential approval of the drug,.

> At the conference, researchers ... presented some of their latest results. They used a clinically validated scale that assesses PTSD symptoms such as frequency of nightmares and anxiety levels. More than one year after two or three sessions of MDMA-assisted therapy, about 67% of participants no longer had the illness, according to that scale. About 23% of the control group — who received psychotherapy and a placebo drug — experienced the same benefit (Maxmen 2017).

At the same conference, Dr Mithoefer presented a video of a former US marine sharing his experience with the MDMA treatment. His explanation is spot on;

> During his conference presentation, Mithoefer [a psychiatrist and clinical researcher] played a video of a former US marine under the influence of MDMA recounting the time his military jeep exploded during a tour in Iraq. The soldier, positioned on a narrow bed between Mithoefer and his wife Annie, a psychiatric nurse, describes the panic that accompanies his memories. But then, he says, an inner-voice assures him that he'll be all right. "I feel things come up and then blow away like sand," the marine says (Maxmen 2017).

The marine went on to say that the effect had lasted and that he and the doctor were still in touch.

PART. B. HOW MDMA WORKS

> [MDMA] also increases levels of certain hormones, including oxytocin and prolactin... Increased levels of oxytocin make people more inclined to connect with others. Oxytocin has also been shown to affect how people respond to certain facial expressions ... research has shown that people given oxytocin are less likely to

> interpret certain facial expressions as being angry or
> threatening…This can be helpful in therapy, particularly
> for people with PTSD, who tend to be hypervigilant and
> looking for threats… oxytocin may allow someone to be
> more trusting (Miller 2017).

MDMA also decreases activity in the amygdala, the place that is responsible
for fear and is overactive in a patient with PTSD.

> The amygdala is the reason we are afraid of things outside
> our control. It also controls the way we react to certain
> stimuli, or an event that causes an emotion, that we see as
> potentially threatening or dangerous (Brain Made Simple
> 2017).

PART C. MDMA AND SEROTONIN SYNDROME

While psychotropic drugs with prescriptions from doctors cause
Serotonin Syndrome, the devastating syndrome I experienced and that is
responsible for most bipolar diagnoses today (according to SSRI Stories
2017) MDMA on its own, does not do this. And it rarely causes side effects
that last

> On its own, MDMA produces feelings of euphoria and
> connectedness, decreasing activity in the amygdala, a
> region of the brain associated with the fear response, and
> increasing activity in the pre-frontal cortex, where higher-
> level brain processing occurs (Ferry 2017).

I would add that the other two hormones released in MDMA, prolactin
and oxytocin (Miller 2017), would stop any drive to take something else. So
it actually safeguards itself against serotonin syndrome in that way.

I am not ready to back the use of MDMA at all. But I can say and will
always say that MDMA helped me immensely. It let me see everything as
malleable. It gave me the ability to dream again and to realize that all of the
trauma was meant to be in order for me to be where I was that night in
Nathan Phillips Square. It allowed me to feel alive again and to not only, in
the weeks and months later, process things that had happened, but to also
make decisions that would ultimately benefit me.

It saved my life.

Today, I don't even drink alcohol and I wonder why I ever did in the
first place. I have no need for it and am never drawn toward drinking or
doing drugs because I don't need them.

It makes me wonder if all of those times in high school and through college where I drank and blacked out were driven by the medications. I started drinking at the same time I was prescribed my first psychotropic drug. Once I stopped the psychotropic drugs, it would not be even two years before I stopped drinking altogether. And not by force. It is now three years past that time.

APPENDIX K

SSRIS, ALCOHOL, ALCOHOLISM AND CRAVINGS

PART A. SEROTONIN AND ALCOHOLISM

> Some of the most commonly prescribed antidepressants are called reuptake inhibitors. What's reuptake? It's the process in which neurotransmitters are naturally reabsorbed back into nerve cells in the brain after they are released to send messages between nerve cells. A reuptake inhibitor prevents this from happening. Instead of getting reabsorbed, the neurotransmitter stays — at least temporarily — in the gap between the nerves, called the synapse (WebMD 2016).

SSRIs cause an influx of serotonin. Alcohol causes a short-lived influx of serotonin. Serotonin Syndrome is caused by too much serotonin building up in the body. Do you see where I am going here?

Check out the conclusion of a study completed in 1997 regarding the role serotonin plays in alcohol abuse:

> Serotonin is an important brain chemical that acts as a neurotransmitter to communicate information among nerve cells. Serotonin's actions have been linked to alcohol's effects on the brain and to alcohol abuse. Alcoholics and experimental animals that consume large quantities of alcohol show evidence of differences in brain serotonin levels compared with nonalcoholics. Both short- and long-term alcohol exposure also affect the serotonin receptors that convert the chemical signal produced by serotonin into functional changes in the signal-receiving cell. Drugs that act on these receptors alter alcohol consumption in both humans and animals. Serotonin, along with other neurotransmitters, also may contribute to alcohol's intoxicating and rewarding effects, and abnormalities in the brain's serotonin system appear to play an important role in the brain processes underlying alcohol abuse (DM 2017).

Alcohol increases serotonin levels in the short term and if you are on a SSRI, it would only make sense that your serotonin levels would skyrocket, sending you into Serotonin Syndrome, where you engage in risky behaviors and act manic. This is also why people would experience "blacking out." The overload sends your nervous system into overdrive. Then, because of the way alcohol works, there is a dramatic drop in serotonin levels, and you would suffer an intensified hangover, one that, if you are already depressed, may cause you to take action when you would not have otherwise.

I think it is fair to say, with such a dramatic fluctuation in serotonin levels, and having hit ecstasy with Serotonin Syndrome, a person might well reach for alcohol when they experience a drop in serotonin levels in order to get back to where they were mentally. In fact, their body may physiologically crave serotonin and cause the person to crave alcohol.

Drug companies would never want drinking to be in the way of their sales, so they don't warn patients in regard to this phenomenon.

> There is an alarming connection between alcoholism and the various prescription drugs that increase serotonin. The most popular of those drugs are PROZAC, ZOLOFT, PAXIL, LUVOX, SERZONE, EFFEXOR. For seven years, numerous reports have been made by reformed alcoholics (some of whom have been sober for fifteen years and longer) who feel "driven" to alcohol again after being prescribed one of these drugs. And many other patients who had no previous history of alcoholism have continued to report an "overwhelming compulsion" to drink while using these drugs (Tracy).

Tracy references a scientific study performed in 1994 on a new antidepressant drug, m-Chlorophenylpiperazine [MCPP] that works with the neurotransmitter serotonin.

> m-Chlorophenylpiperazine produced ethanollike effects and alcohol craving in recently detoxified alcoholics … These data further implicate serotonergic systems in the discriminative properties of ethanol and may indicate a serotonergic contribution to craving (Krystal 2017).

PART B. PROBLEMATIC BEHAVIOR, DEVELOPING A CRAVING

There are several articles about extremely problematic behavior developing as SSRI treatment commenced. The scary part was that below the articles, multiple people commented that the drug did the same thing to them.

One man was put on an SSRI following the death of his father.

> I began to get into trouble with the police, in the main for continual nuisance phone calls to the police station. This happened on a regular basis when I was drinking. Sometimes I would ring them 20 to 30 times a night on their non-emergency number with only a very vague memory of doing so. It resulted in me getting arrested on numerous occasions … (Healy 2017).

The article then explains he developed cravings for alcohol.

> I got cravings for alcohol that were so intense I felt I was possessed. I would start drinking and couldn't stop. I'd continue until I was either arrested or I collapsed into a coma. (Healy 2017).

I was looking for evidence of the insanity that ensued after my drug roller coaster and found that many people had the same story.

Outside of the internet, my mother has come to me with two stories of adult women who were put on certain medications after a loss of a parent.

One of her clients found herself on the roof of a building without any memory of getting there. She had been in the hospital for months after falling. She says she had just been put on medication to treat her depression and that before the medication she couldn't get out of bed. But then this happened. She had no intention of jumping; she had kids at home and was more baffled by how she got up there.

Another woman met her husband, thank God, after drinking and blacking out while taking a common antidepressant. She said that her friends reported extremely strange behavior and that they lost her not long after she started drinking. She woke up extremely on the tile floor on some person's bathroom, having no recollection of the night before. She ended up marrying the man who owned the house and took care of her that night. Obviously, that type of blessing doesn't happen often.

> The serotonin transporter gene has been linked to excessive drinking, early-onset problem drinking, alcohol dependence, anxiety and impulsiveness. While the evidence for antidepressant use appears consistent in alleviating depressive symptoms in patients with comorbid alcohol dependence and depression, some groups of patients may show an increase in alcohol consumption.

Alternatively, there are a series of studies suggesting that antagonism of S-3 receptors can lead to diminished cravings for alcohol (Atigari 2017).

APPENDIX L

ALCOHOL AND MENTAL HEALTH

It is no secret that alcohol can have a detrimental effect over time and if used with abandon. But here are a few statistics regarding alcohol use.

> Nearly 30% of Americans have a problem with alcohol at some point in their lives, ranging from binge drinking to full-blown alcoholism. Excessive alcohol consumption can contribute to learning and memory problems, poor performance at school or work, and mental health problems including depression and anxiety (Alban 2017).

If this is true then this is one more thing to look at when scanning my history and my current state. Alcohol is a depressant widely known for causing damage short and long term to the user. Mental health problems like anxiety and depression as well as dependence are reported. When I do the math it seems like a really bad joke. If these psychotropic drugs are causing alcohol craving and then in turn the alcohol cravings cause mental health issues and on top of that, the depressed or anxious patient looks for a third thing to help the pain, you've got the ingredients of a PTSD smoothie. And yet, not once was I warned about taking these drugs with alcohol.

Fortunately our brains have the ability to heal themselves. The term neuroplasticity has been thrown around a lot recently and for good reason. Neuroplasticity is the ability our brain has to change over time.

> Even when alcohol abuse has altered the size, structure and function of the brain, the damage can be reversed surprisingly fast. After just one day of alcohol abstinence, some increase in gray matter can be detected. After only two weeks of abstinence, the brain measurably increases in volume leading to significantly better cognitive function. Long periods of alcohol abstinence can restore even a heavy drinker's brain back to normal (Alban 2017).

APPENDIX M

HOW ANTI-EPILEPTIC DRUGS WORK

> The way AEDs work is not fully understood. How AEDs have been developed is somewhat 'random' either by luck (finding that an existing drug used for something else happens to work on seizures), or by huge numbers of different drugs being tried in an effort to find one that works (Epilepsy 2017).

Well that sounds about right…

There are a few different types of antiepileptic drugs, but they all work by disrupting the way the brain receives and then interprets certain information. Just as any other oral medication. After the pill is ingested, the digestive juices go to work and the medication passes through the wall of the gut into the bloodstream. The bloodstream takes the medication to the intended area.

AEDS go to the brain.

Hold up, though, once they arrive at the brain, they encounter a blood-brain barrier that prevents things from easily crossing into the brain. This system protects your brain from toxic chemicals and infections.

Drugs do not pass easily through the blood-brain barrier, and for good reason! It's like a shield. But, although the brain has a good enough supply of blood pumping into it, the process in which the medicine actually gets into the brain depends on how well the medication is able to pass through that barrier.

> Some AEDs are not metabolised, not affected by hepatic enzymes and they are excreted in the same form in the urine (Epilepsy 2017).

This is quite possibly the reason for my diagnosis of a fatty liver at one point in college and also the recurrent kidney stones that follow me through college and into audio engineering school.

PART B. TARGETS FOR AEDs

> AEDs may affect the neurotransmitters responsible for sending messages, or attach themselves to the surface of neurones and alter the activity of the cell by changing how ions … flow into and out of the neurones (Epilepsy 2017).

There are four targets for AED medication:

1. SODIUM CHANNELS

> Sodium channels affect how 'excitable' neurones are and how easily messages are sent from one brain cell to another (Epilepsy 2017).

2. CALCIUM ION CHANNELS

> Calcium channels are particularly involved with sending a message from one neurone to another, by affecting the release of neurotransmitters across the synapse. (Epilepsy 2017).

3. GABA SYSTEM AND RECEPTOR AGONISTS

> GABA is a type of inhibitory neurotransmitter in the brain, which effectively stops brain messages from continuing to be sent … Increasing the making of GABA, reducing its breakdown, and increasing its movement, all result in increasing its inhibitory effect (more GABA means more prevention of messages being sent (Epilepsy 2017).

4. GLUTAMATE RECEPTOR ANTAGONISTS

> Glutamate is a type of amino acid, and is a major excitatory neurotransmitter in the brain … Messages are sent from one neurone to another in excitation, due to the movement of sodium and calcium ions into cells, and potassium out of cells … This movement of ions through the cell membranes is helped by glutamate … Drugs that effect and prevent glutamate uptake (antagonists) prevent glutamate from helping the movement of ions through the cell membrane and so prevent the spread of the messages from one neurone to another (Epilepsy 2017).

APPENDIX N

VALPROIC ACID, SEROTONIN (5-HT) AND DOPAMINE (DA)

Depakote's scientific name is valproic acid or divalproex sodium.

Recent studies not only show that valproic acid's efficiency in preventing recurring mania is no greater than a sugar pill, they also show that the medication increases levels of serotonin and dopamine in animal brains. And "few studies have attempted to examine such effects in humans" (Delva 2017).

Let's review what these two very important neurotransmitters, 5-HT and DA, are responsible for:

> Serotonin mediates many physiologic processes and appears to be involved in the pathogenesis of depression, mania, migraine and myoclonic epilepsy, among other conditions ... Altered DA function has also been implicated in several neurologic and psychiatric illnesses, and there is evidence that it is involved in the pathogenesis of mania. ... There is clearly a need for more data on the impact of valproate treatment on serotonergic and dopaminergic neurotransmission in human. (Delva 2017).

This would implicate antiepileptic medications, like Depakote, in causing the symptoms they are prescribed to treat, including migraines and mania. The neurotransmitters responsible for increasing the conditions they were supposed to treat! This would be terrible since the reasons I was prescribed medications varied. When one condition ceased, the doctors keep prescribing the same medication for a new thing.

For example, I was given Topamax for headaches, but at some point the doctor started saying it was for mania.

Depakote was the last psychotropic drug I was prescribed and it was given to me for epilepsy! When I questioned the prescription of the antiepileptic, the doctor reported that it was also used for mania and headaches. I had a stroke due to NuvaRing! I didn't have epilepsy! Ever! But that wasn't even the reason I was prescribed Depakote. Depakote was given to me as a mood stabilizer because of my past.

APPENDIX O

GABAA RECEPTORS AND ALCOHOLISM

PART A. ALCOHOL AND THE GABAA RECEPTOR

> GABAA receptors are also the molecular targets for benzodiazepines and anesthetic barbiturates, both of which share neuropharmacological properties and show cross-tolerance and cross-dependence with alcohol (Paul 2017).

This is frightening because what I am interpreting is that the medications that are given out to treat anxiety, depression, epilepsy and sleep disorders, potentially create a sort of GABA (aka GABAA) mess when mixed with one another.

People should not smoke cigarettes and wear nicotine patches because it makes them ill. They should also not take Suboxone and Norcos because it will make them sick.

> Scientists … now know that there are particular cells in the brain that alcohol targets …The GABA receptor is one of these. Alcohol is an indirect GABA agonist…. Alcohol is believed to mimic GABA's effect in the brain, binding to GABA receptors and inhibiting neuronal signaling. Alcohol also inhibits the major excitatory neurotransmitter, glutamate, particularly at the N-methyl-d-aspartate (NMDA) glutamate receptor…
> it is most likely that the GABA and glutamate receptors in some of the reward centers of the basal forebrain—particularly the nucleus accumbens and the **amygdala**—create a system of positive reinforcement (Scripps 2017).

If antiepileptic medications work as GABA agonists and/or glutamate receptor antagonists as well, [Depakote also generates serotonin and dopamine] isn't there a bit too much happening in the central nervous system.

If someone is drinking and also taking an antiepileptic I would think there would be a compounding effect at the GABA receptors and a compounding inhibitory effect on the NMDA glutamate receptor.

PART B. LIGHTING UP THE BRAIN'S STRESS RESPONSE

> Dependence to alcohol is linked to the interaction of alcohol with the brain's stress system, which alcohol activates. The major component of the brain stress system is the corticotropin-releasing factor (CRF) in the amygdala which activates sympathetic and behavioral responses to stress. … Alcohol interacts in such a way as to acutely reduce CRF levels in the brain; chronic alcoholism does the opposite (Scripps 2017).

If antiepileptic drugs are inhibiting the function of GABA receptors just as alcohol does, and as stated above, light up the amygdala and produce a sort of "reward center," isn't there an issue here with antiepileptics adding to this effect? They are both working on the same neurotransmitter binding site.

> Unfortunately, CRF and the stress system adjust to the alcohol. CRF is hypothesized to persist at artificially high levels in the brain while reward neurotransmitters are compromised (Scripps 2017).

It would seem that this is actually what an antiepileptic is doing to treat someone who does not have seizures. Wouldn't daily use of AEDs then cause the same stress response in the body, since it is working on and in the same way as alcohol within the GABA receptor channel?

Once again, if antiepileptics are working on the same neurotransmitter binding sites, the ones that deal with positive reinforcements and potential for tolerance isn't there an issue here?

> In alcoholism, the effect … results in an equilibration of neurotransmitter levels at artificial … set-points … driven by chronic alcohol ingestion. In the absence of alcohol, the alcoholic feels ill because his or her body cannot easily reverse these artificial levels (for example, high CRF and low reward neurotransmission). When a person overdrinks, there is depleted GABA function in the brain and also, possibly, a hyper-excitable glutamate system (Scripps 2017).
>
> The similarity between the actions of ethanol and sedative drugs such as benzodiazepines and barbiturates that enhance GABA action suggests that ethanol may exert some of its effects by enhancing the function of GABAA receptors (Olsen 2017).

If the AEDS behave the way alcohol does in the brain's stress system, it would cause the potential for addiction by creating the same neurotransmitter suck in which the user would get a rush of CRF levels in the short term and suffer due to the chemical-induced levels of the short-term.

The GABAA receptor is targeted in treatment for epilepsy and by association targeted in whatever case these drugs are prescribed.

APPENDIX P

GABAA and NMDA's Roles in Blackouts

PART A. HOW BARBITUATES WORK

When barbiturates bind to the GABA channel they let more CL-ions into the cells of the brain due to the prolonged opening of the channel. The result of the influx of negative ions is an increased negative charge in the brain cells. This alters the voltage of the brain cells and makes them resistant to nerve impulses (Mandal 2017).

PART B. BLACKOUTS GABAA AND NMDA

> The formation of memory involves … encoding, the initial registration and interpretation of stimuli; storage, consolidation and maintenance of encoded stimuli; and retrieval, which is the search and recovery of stored stimuli.
> Alcohol's effect on encoding may disrupt the processing of context for the formation of an episodic memory. Because the episode was encoded with faulty context, free recall of this memory may be particularly difficult or, depending on the degree of encoding impairment, even impossible, as in the case of en-bloc blackouts.
> In a fragmentary blackout … reminding a subject of events during the blackout often brings on more forgotten memories … giving access to memory that was deficiently encoded.

The trouble encoding memories seems to fit very well with the trouble I had remembering things while taking these medications sans alcohol. The cueing aspect as well as the en-bloc blackouts are eerily familiar.

> In humans, hippocampal damage results in profound impairments in episodic memory with relative preservation of other functions in a way that is remarkably similar to an episode of an alcoholic blackout. …
> One leading candidate for a cellular substrate of memory formation is long-term potentiation (LTP), which is the

establishment of long lasting heightened responsiveness to signals from other cells.

Alcohol inhibits establishment of LTP by potently antagonizing NMDA receptor activity. The NMDA receptor is necessary for LTP induction in area CA1 of the hippocampus. Ethanol's effect on LTP in area CA1 of the hippocampus is thought to involve both inhibition of the NMDA receptor and potentiation of the GABAA receptor transmission, which leads indirectly to further NMDA receptor inhibition (Lee 2017).

It seems to me that the medications I was taking were acting like alcohol to my brain in this sense. They were working on the same neurotransmitters and receptors. So I hypothesize that if I were to drink while taking these meds, blacking out would happen more easily since I was already walking around in a mild blackout state.

APPENDIX Q

DRUG-INDUCED BLACKOUTS [FROM BOOK 1 AND 2]

Throughout high school I blacked out. It became inevitable. No matter what I did, if I drank, at some point in the night, I would lose consciousness mentally, yet appear conscious outwardly.

It was like watching a movie where the film plays without issue right up until a certain point and then the screen suddenly goes completely black: no picture or sound. You wait and wait for the movie to pick back up where it left off, but instead, the film flickers back for a moment, but the scene is blurry, and the characters are now in a completely different time and place than they had been when the screen turned black. Then, before you can sort out what is going on or how the characters got to this new place and time, the screen goes black once more.

Often I would learn that I did mortifying things. It wasn't that I just said embarrassing things, because that is a given drunk-person attribute. I would do things that normal drunk people would never attempt. I heard from different people at various times that at a certain point in the night (usually coinciding with when my memory went dark) my eyes changed. They started to look "vacant."

"You weren't looking back at me. You were, but not really," they would try and explain before shaking their heads. "It was weird; it wasn't you. You didn't look the same."

I attributed these blackouts to the amount of liquor I consumed. And since I don't drink at all anymore, I don't really need to find the answer. But I have strong intuition about this now because many times people did not believe that I had blacked out because they drank just as much as I did or because, they told me, "You didn't even drink that much!" It is very difficult to explain blacking out to a teenager. Most of the time they think you are exaggerating to look cool.

I stumbled across an article about blackouts while researching drug side effects and the definition was spot on for what I experienced countless times.

> A blackout is a period of time where a person is conscious, but is unable to recall any of the events, situations or experiences afterward. A blackout is not passing out, as passing out means you are unconscious. During periods of blackouts, people engage in wild, thoughtless behaviors

that they would not typically engage in otherwise (Newlifeoutlook 2017).

My curiosity, for no specific reason, leads me to search the name of the antidepressant I was taking before the first blackout of this book, alongside the words: "blackout" and "alcohol."

The results are staggering.

I am entranced. I continue down the list of drugs, searching each drug I had been prescribed next to the word "blackouts." I find numerous blog posts of worried individuals wondering if anyone else experiences blackouts while taking [insert antidepressant here] and drinking. Prozac, specifically had over five hundred documented cases of blacking out on one webpage alone (Treato 2016).

Among the list of medications that popped up with significant references to blackouts:

- Prozac
- Lamictal
- Zoloft
- Wellbutrin
- Lyrica
- Effexor

Check out what an attorney says about dealing with his DUI-DWI cases recently:

> As a criminal defense attorney, I see hundreds of clients annually who obtain medications from their physician for anxiety, sleep disorders or depression, yet are not warned to consume NO ALCOHOL when taking these medications. The synergistic effects caused by combining ANY amount of alcohol and these drugs can be devastating for the patient who is surprised to find himself or herself in jail for DUI-DWI, or even vehicular homicide. Blackout, seizures or major amnesia episodes are common. Effexor is currently involved with three of my clients, with others using various common SSRIs and benzodiazepines (Head 2016).

When I tried to find the link that this attorney put in the body of his post, it was broken. I searched the title of his post, "Failure to Warn about SSRIs and Alcohol" and still, nothing. This continually occurred when I tried to access intriguing articles about what patients had experienced while taking certain prescriptions. The links were always broken or the page had been taken down completely.

This happenstance finding of drug-induced blackouts led me to several topics that are truly mind-blowing, including the fact that Serotonin Syndrome actually causes blackouts. And, that blackouts happen in mentally ill people without any substances consumed at all. And the most shocking, that it has been known for a while now that serotonin plays a key role in alcohol craving, dependence and abuse.

It seems pretty obvious to me that if serotonin causes risky behavior and alcohol cravings, it probably causes cravings for other drugs as well. It is like flipping on the switch of addiction in individuals who are already weakened by their diagnosed mental disorder. For example, with no history of personal alcoholism or alcoholism in the family, someone taking a serotonergic drug (any of the SSRIs) would be automatically prone to craving alcohol. (See Appendix K.)

APPENDIX R

HARASSMENT IN THE WORKPLACE

As our new president brought to the forefront of the media, sexual harassment in the workplace is running rampant in our society. One in three women has been sexually harassed at work, according to a recent survey (Vagiones 2017). And it really isn't that hard to believe. Frat boys and sorority girls grow up to be adults in the workforce, and if they were never taught to have empathy for one another, we can't expect it to change. Let's fix this mess.

> … hotlines for reporting harassment are rarely designed to be used by employees. What they're mainly designed for is legal cover for companies, which can point to them, should the need arise … according to Ramona Paetzold, a management professor at Texas A&M University's Mays Business School. 'It is common to have hotlines, to encourage employees to use them, and to make the phone numbers obscure.' (Kessler 2017).

It is fortunate that the awareness has been raised, but now it is time to reform this system. I know I certainly would not feel that calling a hotline of the company I worked at would confidentially and sympathetically assist me in getting out of an uncomfortable situation.

As part of, or at least employed by, the company I was having an issue at, I would reason that, at the end of the day, their job is to assist the company: not me.

GLOSSARY OF USEFUL TERMS

AED: Antiepileptic drug

Black Box Warning: A warning placed on a prescription drug label that is encased in a black box outline to call attention to "serious or life-threatening risks" (FDA 2016).

Chronic Stress Syndrome: a complex form of PTSD (post-traumatic stress syndrome).

Hyponatremia: Low sodium in the blood, can be fatal and cause confusion and psychosis.

Interstitial Cystitis (IC): A chronic, painful bladder condition, and as it turned out, a faulty diagnosis for me. I had kidney stones caused by Topamax.

Serotonin Syndrome (SS): "A life-threatening condition caused by having too much Serotonin in the body" (AAFM 2010).

> "This syndrome consists of a combination of mental status changes, neuromuscular hyperactivity, and autonomic

hyperactivity. Serotonin Syndrome can occur via the therapeutic use of serotonergic drugs alone, an intentional overdose of serotonergic drugs, or classically, as a result of a complex drug interaction between two serotonergic drugs that work by different mechanisms" (Volpi-Abadi et. al. 2013).

SSRI: Selective Serotonin Reuptake Inhibitors, a type of antidepressant that inhibits the absorption of the neurotransmitter serotonin, e.g. Prozac (Ferguson 2001).

Suicidality: Likelihood of an individual to commit suicide (The Free Dictionary 2016).

REFERENCES

The United States Justice Department. "Abbott Labs To Pay $1.5 Billion To Resolve Criminal & Civil Investigations Of Off-Label Promotion Of Depakote". 2017. Justice.Gov. https://www.justice.gov/opa/pr/abbott-labs-pay-15-billion-resolve-criminal-civil-investigations-label-promotion-depakote.

Atigari OV, et al. 2017. "New Onset Alcohol Dependence Linked To Treatment With Selective Serotonin Reuptake Inhibitors. - Pubmed - NCBI". *Ncbi.Nlm.Nih.Gov.* https://www.ncbi.nlm.nih.gov/pubmed/23796469.

The Brain Made Simple."Amygdala - The Brain Made Simple". 2017. Brainmadesimple.Com. http://brainmadesimple.com/amygdala.html.

Drug Dangers. "Depakote - FDA Warning & Legal Information". 2017. Drug Dangers. http://www.drugdangers.com/depakote/.

MedPageToday. "Migraine Drug May Set Stage For Kidney Stones". 2013. Medpagetoday.Com. http://www.medpagetoday.com/meetingcoverage/nkf/38306.

Breggin, Dr. Peter. 2016. "Making A Market In Antipsychotic Drugs: A Tragedy". *The Huffington Post.* http://www.huffingtonpost.com/dr-peter-breggin/making-a-market-in-antips_b_720861.html.

Delva, Nicholas J., Deborah L. Brooks, Brooks, Arun V. Ravindran, Michael Franklin, Khalid Al-Said, Emily R. Hawken, Zul Merali, and J. Stuart Lawson. "Effects Of Short-Term Administration Of Valproate On Serotonin-1A And Dopamine Receptor Function In Healthy Human Subjects". 2017. Pubmed Central (PMC). https://www.ncbi.nlm.nih.gov/pmc/articles/PMC161716/.

Dick, Kirby. *The Hunting Ground*. 2015. Film. Directed By Kirby Dick. Los Angeles: The Weinstein Company.

DM, Lovinger. "Serotonin's Role In Alcohol's Effects On The Brain. - Pubmed - NCBI". 2016. Ncbi.Nlm.Nih.Gov. https://www.ncbi.nlm.nih.gov/pubmed/15704346.

Drobny, Shelby. 2016. "What Drug Companies Are Not Reporting About Alcohol And Anti-Depressants". *The Huffington Post*. http://www.huffingtonpost.com/sheldon-drobny/what-drug-companies-are-n_b_18063.html.

Drugs.Com. "Xanax XR - FDA Prescribing Information, Side Effects And Uses". 2016. Drugs.Com. https://www.drugs.com/pro/xanax-xr.html#PRECdi.

Drugwatch. "Prescription Drug Settlement – Litigation For Dangerous Medication". 2016. Drugwatch. https://www.drugwatch.com/prescription-drug-settlements/.

Epilepsy Society. "How Anti-Epileptic Drugs Work". 2017. Epilepsy Society. https://www.epilepsysociety.org.uk/how-anti-epileptic-drugs-work#.WQfV24n1DdQ.

Ferguson, James. 2016. "SSRI Antidepressant Medications: Adverse Effects And Tolerability". PubMed Central [PMC]. https://www.ncbi.nlm.nih.gov/pmc/articles/PMC181155/.

Ferry, Shaunancy. "FYI: Is Ecstasy Safer When It's Purer?". 2017. *Popular Science*. http://www.popsci.com/science/article/2013-03/fyi-ecstasy-safer-if-its-purer#page-2.

Food and Drug Administration [FDA]. "Suicidal Behavior And Ideation And Antiepileptic Drugs". 2016. Fda.Gov. http://www.fda.gov/Drugs/DrugSafety/PostmarketDrugSafetyInformationforPatientsandProviders/ucm100190.htm.

Food and Drug Administration [FDA]. "A Guide To Safety Terms At The FDA". 2016. FDA.Gov. http://www.fda.gov/downloads/ForConsumers/ConsumerUpdates/UCM107976.pdf.

Food and Drug Administration [FDA]. "Antidepressant Use In Children, Adolescents, And Adults". 2016. Fda.Gov. http://www.fda.gov/Drugs/DrugSafety/InformationbyDrugClass/ucm096273.htm.

Gartlehner, Gerald, Richard Hansen, Ursula Reichenpfader, Angela Kaminski, Christina Kien, Michaela Strobelberger, Megan Noord, Patricia Thieda, Kylie Thaler, and Bradley Gaynes. 2011. "Black Box Warnings Of Drugs Approved By The US Food And Drug Administration". National Center for Biotechnology Information [NCBI]. http://www.ncbi.nlm.nih.gov/books/NBK54348/.

Head, William C. 2016. "Failure To Warn About Ssris & Alcohol". Drugs.Com. https://www.drugs.com/forum/latest-drug-related-news/failure-warn-about-ssris-alcohol-22715.html.

Healy, Dave. 2017. " Driven To Drink: Antidepressants and Cravings for Alcohol". Rxisk.Org. https://rxisk.org/driven-to-drink-antidepressants-and-cravings-for-alcohol/.

Jacqueline Volpi-Abadie, Alan David Kaye. 2016. "Serotonin Syndrome". PubMed Central [PMC]. https://www.ncbi.nlm.nih.gov/pmc/articles/PMC3865832/.

Junger, Sebastian. "How PTSD Became A Problem Far Beyond The Battlefield". 2015. *The Hive*.
http://www.vanityfair.com/news/2015/05/ptsd-war-home-sebastian-junger.

Justice.Gov. "Novartis Pharmaceuticals Corp. To Pay More Than $420 Million To Resolve Off-Label Promotion And
Kickback Allegations". 2016. Justice.Gov. https://www.justice.gov/opa/pr/novartis-pharmaceuticals-corp-pay-
more-420-million-resolve-label-promotion-and-kickback.

Kessler, Sarah. "Corporate Sexual Harassment Hotlines Don't Work. They're Not Designed To". 2017. Quartz.
https://qz.com/971112/corporate-sexual-harassment-hotlines-dont-work-theyre-not-designed-to/.

Khalil Richa S. Thyroid Adverse Effects of Psychotropic Drugs. Clinical Neuropharmacology. 2011;34(6):248-255.
doi:10.1097/wnf.0b013e31823429a7.

Krystal JH, et al. 2016. "Specificity Of Ethanollike Effects Elicited By Serotonergic And Noradrenergic Mechanisms. -
Pubmed - NCBI". Ncbi.Nlm.Nih.Gov. https://www.ncbi.nlm.nih.gov/pubmed/7944878.

Lee, Hamin, Sungwon Roh, and Dai Jin Kim. 2017. "Alcohol-Induced Blackout". Ncbi.Nlm.Nih.Gov.
https://www.ncbi.nlm.nih.gov/pmc/articles/PMC2800062/.

Light of Life Foundation - Light of Life Foundation. Lightoflifefoundationorg. 2016. Available at:
http://www.lightoflifefoundation.org/About-Thyroid-Cancer/About-the-Thyroid-Gland. Accessed July 24,
2016.

Mandal MD, Ananya. 2017. "Barbiturate Mechanism". News-Medical.Net. http://www.news-
medical.net/health/Barbiturate-Mechanism.aspx.

Maxmen, Amy. 2017. "Psychedelic Compound In Ecstasy Moves Closer To Approval To Treat PTSD". Nature:
International Weekly Journal Of Science. https://www.nature.com/news/psychedelic-compound-in-ecstasy-
moves-closer-to-approval-to-treat-ptsd-1.21917.Medchat.com. "Memory Blackouts??? - Medschat". 2016.
Medschat.Com. http://www.medschat.com/Discuss/Memory-Blackouts-178282.htm.

Medshadow. "Drug Classifications, Schedule I, II, III, IV, V - Medshadow". 2016. Medshadow.
http://medshadow.org/drug-classifications-schedule-ii-iii-iv-v/.

Miller, Sarah G. "MDMA For PTSD? How Ecstasy Ingredient Works In The Brain". 2017. Live Science.
http://www.livescience.com/57096-ecstasy-mdma-ptsd-brain.html.

Mundy, Jane. 2017. "Depakote: A Brief History". Lawyersandsettlements.Com.
https://www.lawyersandsettlements.com/articles/drugs-medical/off-label-depakote-birth-defects-00631.html.

New Life Outlook. ""Causes And Treatments Of Bipolar Blackouts". 2016. Newlifeoutlook | Bipolar.
http://bipolar.newlifeoutlook.com/bipolar-blackouts/2/.

Olsen, Richard, and Timothy DeLorey. 2017. "GABA Receptor Physiology And Pharmacology". Ncbi.Nlm.Nih.Gov.
https://www.ncbi.nlm.nih.gov/books/NBK28090/.

Paul, S. M. "Alcohol-Sensitive GABA Receptors And Alcohol Antagonists". 2017. Pubmed Central (PMC).
https://www.ncbi.nlm.nih.gov/pmc/articles/PMC1482489/.

Perry, Dana. *Boy Interrupted*. 2009. Film. Directed by Dana Heinz Perry. HBO Films.

Rachal, Christopher. 2016. "Antidepressant Discontinuation Syndrome - American Family Physician". Aafp.Org. http://www.aafp.org/afp/2006/0801/p449.html.

Ruppe, V. AED-Side-Effects-And-Drug-Interactions. 1st ed. Ferdinand Flynn; 2015. Available at: http://slideplayer.com/slide/4737468/. Accessed July 23, 2016.

Scharff, Ph.D., Constance. "Does MDMA Have Psychotherapeutic Potential?". 2017. *Psychology Today*. https://www.psychologytoday.com/blog/ending-addiction-good/201409/does-mdma-have-psychotherapeutic-potential.

Shuster J. ISMP Adverse Drug Reactions - Hypothyroidism Associated with Quetiapine Therapy; Paradoxical Bronchospasm Associated with Albuterol; Alcohol Cravings with Paroxetine Therapy?; Lamotrigine-Induced Toxic Epidermal Necrolysis – Three Cases; Acute Lung Injury with Vinorelbine; Adverse Events Related to Epinephrine Use in Asthma Patients Seen in the Emergency Department; Collecting Information from Patients Having Adverse Events; New Anticonvulsants – New Adverse Effects. Hospital Pharmacy. 2006;41(7):632-636. doi:10.1310/hpj4107-632.

Smyres, Kerrie. 2017. "Trouble Thinking On Topamax? Study Finds "Language Disturbances"". The Daily Headache. http://www.thedailyheadache.com/2008/02/trouble-thinking-on-topamax-study-finds-language-disturbances.html.

Ssri Stories. "9 Out Of 10 Bipolars Became This Way Through Antidepressant Induced Mania: Doctor Speaks | SSRI Stories". 2016. Ssristories.Org. https://ssristories.org/9-out-of-10-bipolars-became-this-way-through-antidepressant-induced-mania-doctor-speaks/.

Susman, Ed. "Migraine Drug May Set Stage For Kidney Stones". 2013. Medpagetoday.Com. http://www.medpagetoday.com/meetingcoverage/nkf/38306.

Tebb ZTobias J. New Anticonvulsants—New Adverse Effects. *Southern Medical Journal*. 2006;99(4):375-379. doi:10.1097/01.smj.0000209220.40105.0c.

The American Academy of Family Physicians [AAFP]. "Prevention, Diagnosis, And Management Of Serotonin Syndrome". 2016. Aafp.Org. http://www.aafp.org/afp/2010/0501/p1139.pdf.

The American Academy of Family Physicians [AAFP]. "Prevention, Diagnosis, And Management Of Serotonin Syndrome". 2016. Aafp.Org. http://www.aafp.org/afp/2010/0501/p1139.pdf.

The Food and Drug Administration. "Depakote (Divalproex Sodium) Tablets - FDA." 2017. Ebook. 1st ed. The Food and Drug Administration. http://www.accessdata.fda.gov/drugsatfda_docs/label/2011/018723s037lbl.pdf.

The Free Dictionary. "Suicidality". 2016. Thefreedictionary.Com. http://medical-dictionary.thefreedictionary.com/Suicidality.

The United States Department of Justice [DOJ]. "Shire Pharmaceuticals LLC To Pay $56.5 Million To Resolve False Claims Act Allegations Relating To Drug Marketing And Promotion Practices". 2017. Justice.Gov.

https://www.justice.gov/opa/pr/shire-pharmaceuticals-llc-pay-565-million-resolve-false-claims-act-allegations-relating-drug.

Toscano, Amy. 2009. "Depakote Letter-Public Health Service-FDA." Ebook. 1st ed. The Food and Drug Administration. http://www.fda.gov/downloads/Drugs/.../ucm085224.pdf.

Tracy, Ann Blake. 2016. "ICFDA Alcohol Cravings Induced Via Serotonin". Icfda.Drugawareness.Org. http://icfda.drugawareness.org/Archives/Miscellaneous/MRalcohol.html.

UT Southwestern Medical Center. "Drug Prescribed For Migraines And Seizures Increases Risk Of Kidney Stones". 2006. Eurekalert!. https://www.eurekalert.org/pub_releases/2006-10/usmc-dpf102706.php.

Vagiones, Alanna. 2017. "1 In 3 Women Has Been Sexually Harassed At Work". *The Huffington Post.* http://www.huffingtonpost.com/2015/02/19/1-in-3-women-sexually-harassed-work-cosmopolitan_n_6713814.html.

WebMD. "How Different Antidepressants Work". 2016. Webmd. http://www.webmd.com/depression/how-different-antidepressants-work#1.

Welch, Brian J., Dion Graybeal, Orson W. Moe, Naim M. Maalouf, and Khashayar Sakhaee. 2006. "Biochemical And Stone-Risk Profiles With Topiramate Treatment". American Journal Of Kidney Diseases 48 (4): 555-563. doi:10.1053/j.ajkd.2006.07.003.

Welch, Brian J., Dion Graybeal, Orson W. Moe, Naim M. Maalouf, and Khashayar Sakhaee. 2006. "Biochemical And Stone-Risk Profiles With Topiramate Treatment". *American Journal Of Kidney Diseases* 48 (4): 555-563. doi:10.1053/j.ajkd.2006.07.003.

You & Your Hormones | Glands | Thyroid gland. Yourhormonesinfo. 2016. Available at: http://www.yourhormones.info/glands/thyroid_gland.aspx. Accessed July 24, 2016.

Thank You

If you enjoyed the book, please share it with your friends! I very much appreciate your support.

Follow me
for updates, giveaways, inspirational posts, and exciting events to come in the *Finding Kali Trilogy!*

Twitter: @kaliraewheeler

Instagram: @kaliraewheeler

Blog: kaliraewheeler.com

Do you want to get involved?
Have you been through similar experiences?
Please share!
Help me start the discussion on social media with
#findingkali or #findingkalitriology

I'd love to hear your story.
Or
let's get personal!

Visit kaliraewheeler.com
Click "Connect" & send me a message!

Love and Light <3

Namaste,
Kali Rae Wheeler

www.ingramcontent.com/pod-product-compliance
Lightning Source LLC
Chambersburg PA
CBHW032101040426

42336CB00040B/638